Health Adda

demystifying medicine with
chats, insights, anecdotes and
secret prescriptions.

Dr. Gourdas Choudhuri

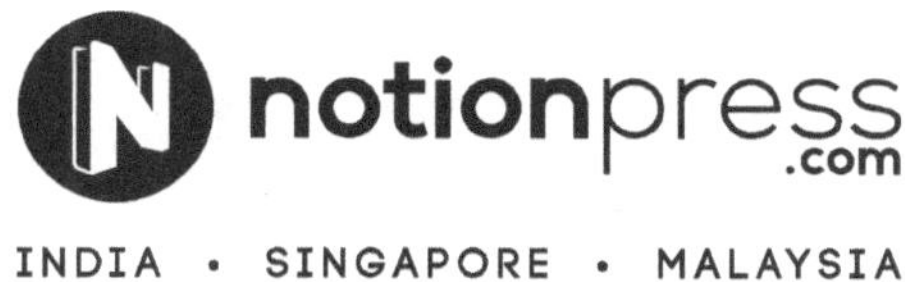

INDIA • SINGAPORE • MALAYSIA

ISBN 979-8-89067-714-3

Books don't just go with you.
They take you where you've never been before.

How to Read This Book

This book can be read at one go, but
I suggest you sip and enjoy it slowly, one or a few chapters at a time.

Sections A, B, C, and D are 'health essentials' to help you survive in modern times, sections F, G, and H will help familiarise you with some common but less talked-about topics, often drawing from the world of news.

Section E deals with common maladies of modern times, some of which either you or someone you know could be afflicted by; topics and chapters here will provide perspectives and insights into recent developments.

Section K takes you to a few boundaries that modern medicine is trying to explore, many of which throw up new challenges to our conventional thinking.

Section L presents to you the human animal in a white coat called 'doctor'.

I hope you enjoy interacting with the book.

Contents

Preface

You're on Earth. There's no cure for that. – Samuel Beckett

Health and disease are 'serious' subjects that you cannot escape in your lifetime. They sometimes float into your mind or infiltrate your conversations. We are somehow so tuned to discuss them in gloomy tones strewn with medical jargon that they chase the casual reader away. In this book, I have tried to discuss these topics in a chatty manner (adda means chat in Bengali language) to engage the general reader.

This is a collection of my short write-ups that appeared as a weekly column called 'Health Adda' since 2009. Several readers relished and enjoyed it and encouraged me to continue writing it for 13 years.

The collection covers a wide range of topics related to 'health' in its broader sense. Grounded in medical science, it takes you through strategies for getting help, our lifestyles and habits, common ailments and cutting-edge research, mindful of the emotions that they generate.

The book does not aspire to be a lighter version of systematic medical text. I have strived to provide perspective and insight on many common health-related topics by adding anecdotes from my experience over the past four decades.

I urge every reader to go through the first four sections for their own good; these will help you get acquainted with common health concerns and apprise you about day-to-day lifestyle issues.

The section on common symptoms and diseases can be like tools in a toolbox; you may look up the ones that concern you or someone in your family from time to time.

The write-ups will come in two sets. This, being the first volume, will introduce you to the physical aspects of lifestyle, health, and some common ailments. The second one will deal with more intriguing aspects of moods, attitudes, and the strange noises that come from our minds while modern science tries to unravel emotions, happiness, and their interplay with our body functions and perceptions.

I wish you an exciting foray into the world of health, medicine, and human life.

Acknowledgement

Had it not been for Sunita Aron, Pankaj Jaiswal, Madhulika Singh, and Deep Saxena, who invited me to write a weekly health column for their paper in 2009 and cheered me week after week, I would not have re-discovered the joy of writing and connecting with general readers. Several readers have urged me to compile them into a book; some of them are Dr. Gautam and Shaswati Palit, Mr.Tajwar Singh Negi, Late Mr. Suresh Gopal (of Bloomsberry), and Mrs. Mridul Chaudhary. Nitika Nagpal enthusiastically put them together. Deepika, Nancy, Glocia and Shreyasi helped in compiling, Indraneil and Tanaya provided critical inputs at various stages.

My daughter Jui, son Deep, and my wife Arundhati showed immense tolerance and support by letting me busy myself on Saturday afternoons writing the next day's column at a prime time that should have been theirs. Their support and suggestions have been a great strength. Arundhati bailed me out by wrapping them up when I was struggling.

My deepest gratitude and salutations are to my patients, who provided deep insights into their health problems, their struggles, challenges and life experiences that have become the best teachers in my medical career. These lessons are unfortunately not found in textbooks, but form the vital link to life, both theirs and mine.

Section A

Gearing Up to Go

In a world of change, the learners shall inherit the earth, while the learned shall find themselves perfectly suited to deal with a world that has ceased to exist.
– Eric Hoffer

01

Google it Right!

Living today requires new and different responses.

If you are one of those who resort to Google or the internet for your health problems, you needn't be embarrassed. You are not the only one. Almost anyone who has access to the internet does it nowadays, either to find out what their symptoms might be indicating or to discover remedies to get better. The inquisitive careful type might go on to learn about illnesses, hunt for the right doctor or hospital, or track his advice and treatment to ensure they are going right.

It is amusing that many doctors are still outraged by the cheekiness of patients trying to cross-check or 'spy' on their 'wisdom', reflecting an outdated attitude of 'paternalistic' medicine.

The internet is a useful repository of information, and in today's world, it is highly unlikely that an average person with a smartphone would not try to discover what it has to offer. It has become an inevitable new factor in patient-doctor relationships.

It is useful, however, not to get confused or frightened by the huge amount of information that it throws at you. Hence, a few basic tips on searching the net, or **Googling it right!** would help.

- Look carefully at the source of the information. What shows up immediately as soon as you type the search words and click the return button are usually advertisements and 'promotional' sites. Most reliable ones would have .edu, .net, or .org after them, indicating that they belong to educational or other reliable organisations. The ones with .com are usually commercial and are likely to be biased.

- If you Google symptoms such as 'constipation', you need to be careful. Most reliable sites will provide a large amount of information and a long list of causes and management. When you go down the list, you will, however, realise that one of the causes listed is cancer of the colon.
- If you put two search terms, such as 'constipation', and a diagnostic term, such as 'colon cancer', most of what will appear on the screen will seem to convey that you might have developed the bad disease. And then starts the anxiety and fear!
- Putting the information in proper perspective, therefore, is the most important bit. For example, if a young person has been suffering from 'constipation' for several years, it is almost invariably going to be due to faulty eating (less amount of dietary fibre, consumption of constipating medicines or food items) or sluggish movement of the colon. If the same symptom occurs for the first time in an elderly person and is associated with rectal bleeding and loss of weight, the chances of the cause being colon cancer go up. This is what the internet does not do well, but the doctor does for you.

ChatGPT is the upgraded version of 'web search' that provides the information that you are seeking. Here again, if your search words and questions are more specific such as "constipation for 6 months in a 20-year-old student staying in a hostel for the last 6 months", then the search results will be much more specific and appropriate for your problem.

- Don't form your opinion based on what you see on social media. These are usually individual opinions, promotional in nature, or reporting of most unusual experiences. If one aggrieved relative posts about the tragic death of his 70-year-old father from cardiac arrest after surgery for colon cancer, you should not believe that that is what usually happens in that situation, just as we do not stop driving on the road because of an accident which happened on the road some time ago.
- The conditions and outcomes posted on social media are often the worst and most unusual ones, as good and happy outcomes are taken for granted and rarely reported.
- Do not hesitate to discuss what you have found on the net with your doctor. He will probably help you navigate through the difficult path and guide you to a balanced clinical decision.
- What the doctor does is run a 'risk versus benefit' calculation in his mind when advising an investigation or procedure. Feel free to ask him about it, but be realistic. Many ask me if I can guarantee a '100-percent-safe' procedure. Well, there is hardly anything that comes with a foolproof guarantee. Driving back home safely from the office without meeting with an accident is also not risk-free.
- The internet may give you all the information, but the doctor can provide his perspective based on experience and knowledge, to guide you in making a balanced decision.

02

Internet, Social Media, and Healthcare

Gentle reminder! You're not too old, and it's not too late.

The internet and social media are impacting medical care in a major way, and trying to stay away from them in today's age when two billion people access them would be archaic. Tuning in to new tools may make life easier for patients and doctors.

Over the last two decades, the internet has come to affect almost every aspect of health care: medical learning, patient-doctor relationships, medical practice, and grievance redressal, to mention a few, and has changed patient behaviour drastically. Those who are tech-savvy and wield a smartphone look up a doctor's or clinic's profile before coming to consult.

Here are five common ways that doctors and patients can use the internet or social media to deliver better care.

1. Scheduling appointments: As the lives of patients and doctors are getting increasingly tight, scheduling an appointment beforehand makes a lot of sense. The website of the hospital or clinic, or the doctor's Facebook page should be able to help you find out where and when to go for consultation and how much it would cost. Taking a day off from work and travelling a long distance to find that the doctor is not available that day can be frustrating. Online appointments and a secretary's cell number can make life much easier.

2. Doctor's details: A doctor's web profile should provide relevant qualifications and professional details so that the patient can choose and decide whom to consult and why. For instance, a patient diagnosed with cancer might want to find out if the doctor is specially trained and experienced in treating that illness.
3. Paid websites and portals often promote doctors, calling some the 'best' and 'greatest' depending on how much has been paid to advertise. Discerning patients, however, get to see through these tricks and seek the 'real' stuff that they need to know. Word of mouth still remains a good tool for confirming a doctor's reputation and capability, especially in small towns. Patients' feedback on the net can offer help too.
4. Educating patients remains a useful method of providing additional care. It helps patients know more about their illnesses, recent progress in the field, and health tips for the family. Nutritional advice, say for heart patients or those with diabetes, can be a good supplement to the consultation.
5. Distraught patients do not usually value insight. Relatives of patients with terminal illnesses are not often comfortable discussing issues surrounding death and dying, preferring the 'fight and blame' approach instead. Dr. Kevin MD's blog deals with larger reflective issues and provide deeper insight for those seeking perceptiveness.
6. The patient-doctor relationship is a two-way interaction and in which the patient has a responsibility too. Doctors should take their feedbacks – providing role honestly. Some patients seek special favours from doctors, such as asking for their personal numbers; if denied, they vengefully write adverse reviews. Reading several reviews from a larger number of patients gives a non-prejudiced clearer picture.

03

Emergency Medical Kit

Chance favours the prepared mind. – Louis Pasteur

The depiction in Indian TV serials of a doctor arriving home immediately when summoned on the telephone to attend to an emergency couldn't be further from reality. Most doctors do not attend home calls, and the chances of getting one in the middle of the night when you are down with an attack of incessant vomiting or an allergy could be almost impossible. Also, for some emergencies, waiting an hour until the doctor arrives may prove costly.

It makes sense, therefore, to keep some medicines at home or carry them on travel. Here are some tips on how to make your own emergency medical kit:

- Keep medicines that you are familiar with, preferably the ones you have taken before. Taking a 'new' medicine for the first time during an emergency without a doctor around, and that too in a new place, is better avoided.
- If you are not good with tongue-twisting drug names, put them in labelled envelopes according to the indications. For example, you could have paracetamol tablets in an envelope labelled 'Fever, Body Pain', or loperamide in one labelled 'loose motions'.
- Keep them in your hand baggage, in a separate pouch or flap.

I recall how a fellow passenger, who had a history of asthma, came down with a severe attack of breathlessness during a long flight from Delhi to Frankfurt. He had remembered to pack his asthma inhalers all right but had put them in the checked-in luggage. Fortunately, the emergency kit of that aircraft had a bronchodilator injection along with a syringe and needle. Having responded to the "Is there a doctor on the flight?" announcement, I had to administer an injection of deriphylline to him mid-air.

- Know your special needs. For example, one who has asthma should ensure he carries bronchodilators, just as one with diabetes should carry not just anti-diabetic medications but also some sweets or sugars in case the head spins due to a drop in blood sugar.
- Consult your family doctor; he will know which medicines are safe and good for you.

The kit could contain medicines to deal with these common emergencies:

- For allergies, hives, itching, running nose, watery eyes, and wheezing: anti-allergic or anti-histamine medications such as Allegra/Alspan/Cetriz/Avil/Monteluk tabs
- For loose motions (watery): loperamide (Imodium)
- For acidity/heartburn: antacid tablets such as digene or gelusil, acid blockers such as Famotidine or PPIs (omeprazole, pantoprazole or rabeprazole)
- For nausea or vomiting: Domperidone or Ondansetron
- For motion sickness: Promethazine (Avomine tablet)
- Traveller's Diarrhoea, watery frequent stools: Rifaximin tablets
- For infections: Tummy or urine infections, fever: Ciprofloxacin or Ofloxacin/ Cephalosporins (like Cetil or Sporidex)
- For throat or chest infections: Cephalosporins, Amoxycillin, or Septran

- For fever, body aches, sprains, and injuries: Paracetamol/Ibuprofen
- For crampy pain in the abdomen or painful periods: smooth muscle relaxants or antispasmodics, such as Spasmindon, Cyclopam, or Meftal Spas
- Also carry a small bottle of nasal drops for a blocked nose (Otrivin), a few medicated Leucoplast (Band-aid) strips, local antiseptic cream (Betadine), a few Oral Rehydration sachets (ORS/ Electral) and laxatives (like Naturolax or Movicol) especially if you are travelling to the West.
- Make sure you have your family physician's cell number at all times
- If you have any medical problem, such as diabetes or blood pressure, carry these medicines in sufficient numbers. Your family doctor will guide you regarding any special medicines that you should keep for your unique needs.

The kit is like the spare tyre that you keep in the car boot on long drives. And there can be a little doctor in each of us to pull us out of unexpected health troubles!

Most of the names of medications suggested are generic or common brand names to help readers procure them easily, after consulting their family doctor.

04

The Good Old GP

To be trusted is a greater compliment than being loved.
– George MacDonald

The family doctor, fortunately, is being resurrected again. Yes, he was almost dead in the last few decades when obsession with specialities and specialists drove patients to high-end tertiary care centres. What they often missed was good holistic care.

The family doctor's role is the most challenging. He has to answer why the newborn cries after feeds, why the school-going child is not eating enough (or at least that is what his mom thinks), why the lady of the house gets the splitting attacks of migraine, how to measure and control the gentleman's BP, why grand-dad takes so long to pass urine, or how to manage the vomiting and diarrhoea of the cousins who are visiting. In other words, he has to be the proverbial jack and dabble with all aspects of health from birth to death.

Being a scarce commodity, a good family doctor can be difficult to find. His qualifications should include more than just the proper degree; he should be easily accessible. He should not be the 'white coat monster' to scare the kids with injections if they don't eat their veggies. He should be accepted more as a family friend whom you can consult for almost anything.

Another essential quality he needs to have is openness. Considering the varied aspects he is questioned on, he should not be expected to know everything about everything (what is a specialist there for?) but should be willing to seek help and guidance from peers, books, or the internet.

Here is a simple test: If he looks irritated with your persistent questions or disapproves of your finding something on the internet about an illness, and gets offended when you bring it up, he is not your guy. On the other hand, if he says he is unsure and needs to read up or consult, go for him.

The family doctor should know the unique aspects of your body system and that of your family: allergies, the painkillers or antibiotics that agree with you, and other medical conditions such as diabetes, hypertension, hypothyroidism, peptic ulcer, proneness to fits or panic (we call them co-morbidities) that often get thrown off-gear during illnesses. And of course your nature or disposition. Treatment or care should ideally be provided keeping all these in mind, an aspect that specialists often tend to overlook.

I find that most patients who go to seek treatment at a speciality centre do not have family physicians. When I specifically ask them to find one near their homes, they appear reluctant and often seem to lack faith in their GPs.

A GP, therefore, needs to reinvent his role and win back the trust of his patients. His steady reassuring presence and ready availability should be his USP. It is he who needs to maintain the balance between over-investigating, aggressive super-specialist's prescribing of strong medications or unproven therapy, and emerge as the medical anchor of the family.

For specialists, patients keep changing, but the diseases remain the same. For family physicians, on the other hand, diseases keep changing while patients remain the same.

05

Finding the Right Doctor can be Tough

The best doctor gives the least medicines. – Benjamin Franklin

Patients planning to undergo major, complicated procedures such as heart surgery, organ transplantation, or joint replacement are often anxious to know about the success rates and risks before making up their minds or choosing the doctor.

Conventionally, it has been word of mouth that guides patients to a particular doctor. "We heard Mr. Sharma, our neighbour's friend, came home well after heart surgery in X hospital by Y surgeon. He must, therefore, be good," is the usual formula.

Another method has been to assess competence by seeing the crowd outside his chamber. This does convey that the doctor is popular, but it could also mean that he is not well organised in managing his clinic crowd.

In this age of computers and the internet, the most common thing smart people do is search the net. This approach, however, could have its own problems.

We are led to believe that more hits on Google mean the doctor is more likely to provide satisfactory treatment. It is, therefore, hardly surprising that corporate hospitals and private doctors have a larger presence on the net than highly skilled specialists in academic and government institutions who did not put any effort into promoting themselves.

Efforts are on in some countries to encourage hospitals and departments to put up data on the internet stating, for instance, how many open heart surgeries have been done, how many have been successful, and how many have succumbed. It is hoped that this kind of transparency will help a prospective patient make a better-informed choice.

Most hospitals and doctors, however, put up only their success stories and touching tales of good outcomes. The endorsement by patients is often preselected to ensure that it is positive giving the gullible browser an impression of great merit that could be far from real.

The genesis of this initiative dates back three decades when a whistle-blower drew attention to an alarmingly high rate of deaths in children undergoing heart surgery in a hospital in England. Now known as the Bristol Heart Case, it was subsequently discovered that 29 of 53 children who had undergone a type of heart surgery at the Bristol Royal Infirmary during a particular period, had died; the mortality rate was an astonishing 55 per cent, much higher than other centres doing similar procedures.

This revelation led to an inquiry conducted by the National Health Services of the UK. Three eminent cardiac surgeons were held responsible for this and were debarred from operating with their names struck off from the council's list.

Indeed, if authentic data about a doctor's experience, success rates, and complications were made available, decision-making for patients would become easier. But with hospitals and specialists competing with each other in marketing, ensuring authenticity of data remains a challenge.

'Word of mouth' or a neighbour's advice will still have a place and be valuable; patients who have had a good outcome are more likely to heap praise, often mixed with gratitude, while relatives of those who failed to make it might be scathing in their feedbacks.

06

What Makes Modern Medicine Modern

Without research, medicine would be an art based on superstition.
- Archie Cochrane

Heart diseases, for instance, can now be prevented by new drugs that lower cholesterol or prevent the stickiness of clot-forming platelets, thanks to research that is providing a steady stream of new medications. Narrowed or blocked arteries of the heart can now be opened up by balloons or have stents inserted across them, thanks again to bold research. Further, the occluded arteries can also be 'bypassed' surgically using grafts or conduits that research and experimentation threw up over 30 years ago.

What has made these advances possible, however, has been years of painstaking research, initially in laboratories, then on animals in labs, and finally on human subjects. And if the terms 'research' and 'clinical trial' evoke creepy feelings of cold, inhuman experimentation, remember that the benefits we enjoy today would not have come otherwise. There must have been the first few who went through these therapies that were experimental then.

As a corollary, the lack of research has made several systems that once had their day in the sun, obsolete. A great Roman physician called Claude Galen lived in the second century CE. His observations and teachings reached historical heights; his potions made from herbs were THE treatment those days. The next hundred years witnessed the blind practice of what Galen had written, with no new research or addition. Progress soon came to a halt, and history now looks back at this period as the Dark Age of Western Medicine. Our Indian systems of medicine, once rich and flourishing, have also been plagued by a lack of new research.

Hepatitis B infection, a leading cause of liver failure and liver cancer that had no remedy till the mid-eighties, now has six good medicines and an effective vaccine for prevention, thanks to medical research. Hepatitis C infection, which had only expensive and toxic injections of interferon by way of therapy till 2014, has now become one of the simplest infections to treat, with simple effective oral drugs taken for just three months. The only way these make it into our arsenal is after research and trials on lab animals, and then patients, to prove that they are effective and safe.

Needless to say, medical research needs to meet high standards of ethics, care, and safety, and be transparent and accountable. Research needs encouragement and promotion too if medicine is to continue its advancement. Banning it would halt its progress and take us back to the Dark Ages.

07

Cures are Rare in Medicine

Life belongs to the living, and he who lives must be prepared for changes. – Goethe

The patient who frightens me most is the one who presents with a decade-long history of symptoms, a thick file of test reports, and multiple prescriptions of several medical consultations and goes on to tell me at the end of his long account that he has come to me to seek a 'cure' that has evaded him all this while.

I usually shudder at that stage of the consultation and find myself unable to decide whether to be brusque and upfront and tell him bluntly that his expectation is unrealistic—an approach that would save his time and mine—or chide along with comforting words and gradually bring him around to accepting that like most diseases such as diabetes, high blood pressure, or hypothyroidism, his problems of acidity and constipation can be 'managed' but not entirely 'cured'.

In fact, Erich Segal's famous novel Doctors opens with an address by the dean to the new students entering Harvard medical school, where he startles the youngsters with the humbling confession that only a handful among the thousands of medical illnesses that we recognise, actually have a true cure; the remaining majority can be just 'managed' or controlled.

Cure usually implies that the problem is eradicated from the body for good and is possible usually with infectious diseases such as typhoid, malaria, tuberculosis, pneumonia, amoebic infections, or hepatitis C, where medications are available to kill the invading germs. It is now possible with some cancers too such as early breast, skin, or uterine cancers, some blood cancers, and some lymphomas. Stones that have formed in the kidney or the gallbladder can be surgically removed permanently, too.

Despite not having specific anti-microbial therapy, some infections are cured by themselves by simply moving out of the body, permitting the host to recover from what is called a 'self-limiting illness'. Examples include the common flu, hepatitis A and E, dengue fever, swine flu, viral diarrhoea, and even viral meningitis. The acute phase may be deadly, but once overturned by the body's own defence mechanisms, the recovery is permanent, satisfying the definition of 'cure'.

Shouldn't these humbling observations make a doctor of modern medicine cringe rather than take pride in belonging to the medical profession?

Well, to start with, keeping diseases under long-term control, even if they are not quite cured, brings significant benefits to life—both in length and quality. Timely detection of high BP, diabetes, thyroid disorders, and hepatitis B has already led to an increase in life expectancy and a reduced risk of heart attacks, stroke, or liver cirrhosis in a large number of people.

Modern medicine is based on evidence-based knowledge enabling doctors to spot illnesses that can be cured in a few, or managed in a majority of cases so that patients can live longer and healthier lives. It is critical to diagnose the few diseases for which modern medicine may not have much to offer and discuss them frankly rather than taking them on an expensive ride.

Modern medicine, while being imperfect, remains an open book and maintains a distinct advantage over its rivals, who often promise a cure to every patient for every illness.

Well, a known devil is better than an unknown saint.

08

How Long Do You Wish to Live? Is Life Expectancy Hitting the Ceiling?

It is not how long you live, but how you live that matters.

The average life expectancy of Indians has climbed steadily over the decades to 70 years. To put it in simple terms, a baby born in India today may be expected to live for around 70 years.

This figure is impressive in several ways. For one, it has doubled from what it was around the middle of the last century. We need to keep in mind that the major contributor has been the reduced number of deaths in infancy and childhood, thanks to the effective national immunisation programmes for infants and children, and the control of infections such as cholera and diarrhoea.

If we look around, we realise that there is still much ground to cover. Most developed industrial nations have life expectancy figures well above 80. In France, for example, the average life expectancy is 85 for women and 79 for men. And the figures are steadily rising.

As of December 2022, the longest-living person in the world, after 119-year-old Japanese woman, Kane Tanaka, who died in April 2022, was 118-year-old French nun, Sister Andre.

The French and the Japanese attribute their long lives to healthy eating, regular exercise, and avoiding bad habits such as smoking. The French, in addition, feel a glass of red wine daily contributes to their health and well-being, which Sister Andre has been consuming from her early days.

Sister Andre had lost her sight and was wheel chair dependent, but was mentally alert. When asked in a TV interview in late 2022, what she wanted most at that stage of her life, she ironically said without hesitation that she just wanted to die.

That brings us to the question: *What do we value more—length of life or good quality of life as long as we live?*

There is no doubt that as life expectancy has increased, people are consciously trying to keep themselves fitter. For instance, the age of 60, which was long considered the time when one retired and receded into old age in an armchair or in bed, is now considered the time when one begins the next phase of life and explores a new occupation or activity.

While the extension of life expectancy is worth the medical efforts, we must also focus on how best to add purpose, enjoyment, and productivity to this phase. Mere prolongation of life in a bedridden, demented state may not always be an attractive option, as Sister Andre mentioned.

Section B

Lifestyle

As long as you live, keep learning how to live. – Seneca

01

Eat Breakfast like a King

Well begun is half done.

"If you skip breakfast frequently or eat very small ones, you might be at risk for developing obesity," say medical scientists. Most people who grow a paunch have often been small breakfast eaters, consuming most of their calories at dinner. Conversely, if dinner is heavy and late, the risk of obesity goes up.

A team of chrono-nutritionists from the Imperial College, London, studied eating patterns across the world and found sense in the old adage—*breakfast like a king, lunch like a prince, and dinner like a pauper.* This scientific branch deals not just with 'what' and 'how much' you eat but also with how the timing of meals influences body metabolism and health.

The review included ten studies that looked at the link between the time of day when one eats and body weight or BMI (Body Mass Index). It revealed that obese people were more often frugal breakfast eaters and large late diners. In fact, the study noted that those who ate large breakfasts maintained a normal weight.

This study also showed significant cultural differences in eating habits and identified four main patterns of food consumption in different countries:

- Equal energy consumption at breakfast and dinner, with the greatest consumption at lunch in Guatemala and Poland.

- Smallest energy consumption at breakfast, greatest consumption at lunch, followed by dinner in France, Switzerland, and Italy.
- Equal energy consumption at breakfast and dinner, with the smallest consumption at lunch in Sweden.
- Smallest consumption at breakfast, greater consumption at lunch, and greatest consumption at dinner in the UK, the US, Germany, Canada, Denmark, the Netherlands, and Belgium.

Most of us in India probably fall into the last category. What further complicates the issue is that we often go to bed soon after our dinner, with very little opportunity to burn off the excess calories consumed at dinner.

Late-large diners have other health problems too, apart from obesity. They suffer from night-time gastro-oesophageal reflux and have troubled sleep. They often wake up at night, choking. Further, as food is not well digested during sleeping hours, bowel movements are also often erratic, causing constipation.

For people who need alert, well-functioning brains, such as students and scholars, a heavy breakfast could help. Studies have shown that glucose supply to the brain in the morning keeps them alert and attentive, thereby facilitating memory and logic. Breakfast skippers, on the other hand, often feel lethargic and sleepy as blood levels of glucose drop during school hours.

A good heavy breakfast should consist of wholegrain cereals, fruits, and proteins (cheese, eggs, and milk) thereby providing a sufficient amount of starch, fats, and proteins. Starch has an important role in breakfast as it is the main supplier of glucose that the brain needs. That is the reason why cereals, cornflakes, and idlis are so popular for this meal.

Parathas for breakfast and *sukhi* roti for dinner may not be a bad idea after all!

02

How Do You like Your Tea?

There is something in the nature of tea that leads us into a world of quiet contemplation of life. – Lin Yutang

The way we drink our tea may reflect not just our taste and style but our health too.

Tea drinking is a 4,700-year-old custom that has its origin in China. The leaves of the shrub Camellia sinensis (tea plant) were used at that time as a remedy for wounds and diseases. With the legendary emperor Shenong brewing and drinking its extracts, tea drinking became a popular habit in this part of the world.

The British, impressed with the brew and the customs that go with drinking tea in China and Japan, tried to emulate and evolve a tea-drinking custom of their own, and soon 'tea-time' became a familiar term across the globe.

Every home or cafe seems to have its own flavour. The north Indian variety of 'chai' is a glass of hot, creamy milk (more cream, more special it is!) with lots of sugar and lacing of strong 'tea liquor' from the tea gardens at lower heights in Assam, Nilgiris, Sri Lanka, etc. In contrast, the Chinese and Japanese prefer light green or jasmine tea without a drop of milk. Some relish the Darjeeling variety that grows at high altitudes; it has a distinct flavour; the liquor is mild and is best consumed with little or no milk.

Tea contains a substance called caffeine (15–50 mg per cup) that boosts mental alertness, increases short-term memory, and has a mild anti-depressant effect; hence, many prefer to have it first thing in the morning to get out of bed, before exams, or when alertness is required.

A special group of healthy substances called antioxidants is abundant in tea, especially the green or jasmine varieties. The antioxidant epigallocatechin gallate (EGCG) has anti-cancer properties; it lowers stress levels, protects the heart, and prevents degenerative diseases like Parkinsonism or dementia. A recent study showed that people who drank two cups of green tea a day had a 50 per cent less decline in mental function with ageing. Not surprisingly, tea-drinking Chinese and Japanese elders often live till 100 while remaining alert till late.

Tea (green or jasmine only, not creamy ones) also boosts our metabolic rate and helps maintain slim figures. Catechin polyphenols and caffeine probably do the trick by increasing the burning of fat in the body. Where tea really scores over coffee is in its glycaemic index, or propensity to push up blood sugar. It is three in green tea compared to 13 in chai and 27 in a cup of coffee. Tea drinking also helps avoid bad breath.

Many are taking to jasmine tea these days. It is a blend of jasmine buds (originally from Persia) with green or white tea and is mild and soothing. Try drinking two to five cups of jasmine tea a day and see how refreshing it makes you feel. There are several other flavours to choose from such as cardamom, orange-pekoe, masala, and more.

Enjoy your cup of tea!

03

Much Can Happen with Coffee

Science may never come up with a better office communication system than the coffee break. – Earl Wilson

The buck-you-up cup that gets us going in the morning has indeed survived intense scientific scrutiny for 20 years regarding its health benefits, has emerged largely unscathed, with some benefits to claim instead. A recent study showed that moderate coffee drinkers were less likely to develop liver cirrhosis, degenerative brain disorders, and heart diseases.

Scientists, still trying to understand the cause of the enigmatic Alzheimer's disease, a degenerative condition of the brain that wipes off its victim's memory and higher mental functions, were surprised to find that those who drank three to five cups of the brew a day had a lower chance of having the disease. A similar 'protection' was also seen in another degenerative condition of the nerves and brain, called Parkinson's disease.

Coffee, a drink made from brewing beans of the Coffea plant, contains several chemical compounds that affect the human system. Apart from caffeine, the main constituent that provides its stimulant effect, it contains a wide range of other substances, antioxidants, and minerals such as zinc, selenium, and copper.

Coffee is widely believed to have originated in the Arabian Peninsula, where its use can be traced back to as early as the 15th century. It was introduced many years later into Europe, the Americas, and the rest of the world. It came to India around the 17th century, when six coffee pods were planted near Mysore. The ensuing cultivation and consumption of coffee in the region saw the ushering in of the 'kapi' culture that is so prevalent in the south.

The short-term effects of the drink are well known: it stimulates the brain, helps fight sleep, and increases urination. Overstimulation may cause anxiety, sleeplessness, palpitations, a rise in blood pressure, and increased blood sugar levels through the release of stress hormones—epinephrine and cortisol. The risk of stillbirth may increase if coffee is consumed excessively during pregnancy, and one may suffer from anaemia due to coffee interfering with the absorption of iron in the gut.

Studies, however, show a protective effect against a variety of diseases among regular and moderate coffee drinkers. They are less likely to develop gallstones, dental caries, and gout, and also have a low risk of suffering from heart disease, hypertension, migraine, and diabetes. Antioxidants in the drink probably account for most of these benefits, as do the minerals selenium and zinc, which protect against diabetes by stimulating the pancreas.

Coffee drinking is churning society too, widening the rift between the classic filter-coffee lover and the new-age young aficionado who can confidently have his pick from the mind-boggling variety that a coffee-bar menu now offers: cappuccino, latte, or expresso; Arabic, Brazilian, or Indian; large, moderate, or small; decaf or normal; hot or iced; with or without sugar, etc.; his nonchalance often assuming a style statement.

Coffee drinking is clearly evolving, offering variety in the type of drink, place, and style for everyone and every occasion. It has found its place in poetry with, "I have measured out my life with coffee spoons," famously introduced by my favourite poet TS Eliot.

How did you have your morning cup?

04

Cooking Medium

In a world of propaganda, truth is always a conspiracy.

Some of my cardiologist friends, who look at my paunch and mischievously ask how my tennis sessions are going, are often at a loss to explain why the last king of Oudh (Awadh), Nawab Wajid Ali Shah, who was very fat and epitomised laziness, lived till his mid-sixties without needing their expensive services of coronary angioplasty or bypass surgery.

The Nawab had quite a few patently obvious health risks. Pictures show him as being grotesquely obese, and his 'nawabi' laziness has been legendary. He is said to have been so dependent on his servants that he could not put on his shoes by himself. He could not waddle out of his palace by himself to escape the British soldiers when they reached his palace, as his servants had fled and he was shoeless.

Plump people who do not exercise regularly are usually fond of food, as His Royal Highness was. He is said to have instructed his cooks to change the cooking medium (probably ghee) to fry his royal *parathas* (stuffed fried bread) with an abundant helping of fresh ghee for each side.

On hearing this tale, I got the uncanny feeling that the nawab's cardiologists would have intuitively tipped the nawab that reheating the cooking medium could be harmful to his heart. How else could he, in the 18th century, possibly know that oils and fats, which exist in their *cis*-chemical form in their natural state, change to *trans* fats when heated repeatedly? Modern cardiologists swear by their dangling stethoscopes that these *trans* fats, regardless of their sources and backgrounds, arise from the reheating of fats and oils, and are notorious for getting deposited and clogging the arteries of our hearts.

This vital health tip somehow got obscured in the next two hundred years until the coronary arteries of the smart-figured, energetic American president Bill Clinton clogged, necessitating two surgeries to restore blood flow to the crying muscles of his choking heart in 2004. Mind you, he was neither fat nor lazy, unlike the nawab.

Mr. Clinton's fondness for food was as legendary as that of the Nawab. He admits to gorging passionately on fast food and hamburgers for most of his pre-heart surgery life. Once, on an aerial survey of a disaster-hit region, he is believed to have seen the Big Mac's M and cheered, "Hey, we will get burgers here!"

What possibly made all the difference to their hearts was the amount of *cis*-fats in the parathas that the nawab ate and the *trans* fats in the chips and burgers the American president consumed.

If *samosas* and *jalebi* are something you can't do without, get them from your *halwai* in the morning when he has started the day with a fresh supply of oil. Come evening, and after several sessions of frying and reheating, the concentration of *trans* fat shoots up enormously, making them toxic to the heart.

Homemakers who pray for their husbands' health and longevity would do well to use lesser quantities of oil, fry shallow rather than deep, and change the oil frequently when frying *puris* or *samosas* for their beloved husbands.

05

Sugar Addiction and Fatty Liver

You become so close to your addictions and illnesses that leaving them behind is like killing the part of yourself that taught you how to survive. – Lacey L

The word 'addiction' brings to mind alcohol, tobacco, and psychotropic drugs. But sugar is emerging as a new addiction that we might be ignoring and passing off as just an innocent fancy.

Many of us describe ourselves as having a 'sweet tooth' and indulge our taste buds and liver with excess sugar.

In several scientific conclaves on fatty liver disease, doctors now report how addiction to sugar and sugary drinks has emerged as a major cause for concern in the last few decades.

Statistics are worrying. Several Indian hepatologists report excess fat in the livers of up to 50 per cent of Indians, especially those living in cities. The BMI of urban school children has been rising, with over 30 per cent now being overweight. And what seems to be the common denominator is excess consumption of sugar through sweets, fruit juices, and pastries.

Addiction to sugar is now established. Those suffering from it show all the typical symptoms, from regular 'wants', to increasing demands, to desperate needs or cravings. If one is to go without sweets for a day or two, he shows anger and irritability that withdrawal is known to be associated with.

A special subset of sugar addiction is 'fructo-holism'. Fructose is the predominant sugar in fruits and juices, and some people have been found to be addicted to this variety of sugar. Scientists have observed that fructose sugar causes a greater accumulation of fat in the liver, more than what happens with regular sugar—sucrose.

In a chilling account of what we have always considered innocuous and perhaps even healthy, excess fructose has been shown to get converted to fat and deposited in the liver, causing fatty liver.

But why should that worry us? It is now clear that those who have extra fat in the liver are at increased risk of developing the 'metabolic syndrome', a package of excess body weight, diabetes, hypertension, and high blood lipids, all of which confer an increased risk of cardiovascular or heart disease.

Cardiovascular diseases such as heart attack or stroke, and metabolic diseases such as diabetes and hypertension, have emerged as the most common cause (60 per cent) of death and ill health in India. And what might be fuelling them could be our social practices and indulgence in sweets and fruit juices.

It is time we took note and changed our practices and preferences.

06

Microbial Garden in Your Gut

To plant a garden is to dream of tomorrow. – Audrey Hepburn

Scientists are perplexed to come to terms with the observation that germs or small microbes, long-held responsible for causing diseases, could be essential for maintaining the health of the human body. In fact, our body is loaded with germs, over a trillion (10^{14}) in our guts alone, and quite a few residing on our skins and noses too.

They belong to as many as 400 different species. If we could scoop them all out and place them on a weighing scale, they would weigh as much as 1.5–3.0 kg, which is even more than the clothes we wear.

The presence of this huge, bustling wildlife sanctuary of little animals or microbial garden in our gut has puzzled scientists. There was a time when 'germs' were those terrible little things that caused nasty infections and often took lives. In fact, when some of these germs migrate from the gut to abnormal places such as the urinary tract, they produce illnesses such as urine infections.

The logical approach that scientists, therefore, took in the last two centuries, was to rid the body of all germs in an attempt to 'sterilise' it. They soon realised that removing the 'good' germs often cleared the field for disease-producing bacteria to invade the body and cause diseases.

It has now become clear that good germs need our warm, moist, and slushy guts to survive, breed, and colonise, and act as guards preventing bad germs from gaining a foothold and invading the body to cause disease.

The most dramatic example in current times is a condition called 'antibiotic-associated diarrhoea (AAD)' or the upset tummy that many of us experience when we take antibiotics for infections of the throat or lungs.

The gripes and 'loosies' we get are best managed by consuming 'good' germs, called probiotics, either in the form of curd or yoghurt or as preparations that come in the form of capsules or liquids. A particular variety of healthy germs called *Saccharomyces boulardii* has been shown to work best for this condition.

Scientists have now gone a step further. They have taken germs from a healthy person and transplanted them or put them into people with weak guts? Stool transplant, or faecal microbiota transplant (FMT) as it is called, involves taking stools from healthy donors, running them through labs to ensure the absence of harmful germs, and sprinkling them in the patient's intestines through a tube passed from either end of the gastrointestinal tract.

There are several medical centres in the world and a few in India that have started doing FMT. One of the conditions for which FMT has proven to be effective is 'Clostridium Difficile' disease which does not go away easily with medications but responds well when the gut garden is planted with good germs that push out the bad ones. The results of this procedure are thrice as good as any other form of treatment. It is being increasingly tried in a variety of other conditions, such as ulcerative colitis, some forms of liver failure, metabolic diseases such as diabetes, and graft-versus-host disease—an immune disorder that affects some who have undergone bone marrow transplantation.

While many of these indications are in the early stages, initial results are promising.

The Chinese seemed to have known all this as far back as the 4th century BC. They had a practice of young mothers feeding a small bit of their stools to their newborns to make their infants' guts strong.

We have come a full circle now with faecal transplantation to regain our health.

07

Yoga and Health

The body benefits from movement, and the mind benefits from stillness. Yoga is the dance of every cell with the music of every breath that creates inner serenity and harmony.

Yoga means many things to many people: from practising postures or asanas to make the body flexible, to the rhythmic control of breathing and beating of the heart, to focusing our wandering minds and many more.

A Google search of 'Yoga and Health' threw up more than a million hits, many of which were, of course, promotional. When I searched Pubmed for peer-reviewed scientific and medical literature with the same search words, I came across an astonishing 9,000 publications, indicating that yoga has indeed now crossed the road from being a mere antiquated Indian practice to a contemporary health aid well-accepted by modern medicine.

Interestingly, many, if not most, scientific studies on yoga seem to come from the Western world, where scientists and doctors have used modern tools and methods to evaluate its effect on health outcomes.

Yoga has proven to be beneficial in a wide range of non-communicable or lifestyle diseases such as diabetes, high or low blood pressure, some forms of heart disease, increased cholesterol, obesity, fatty liver, backaches, arthritis, and chronic respiratory problems.

Other disorders where it has worked well include slowing down ageing, improving posture and balance, lifting depression, calming anxiety, and improving poor concentration.

Additional feathers that could make yoga more attractive to people are its claims of ameliorating sexual dysfunction and improving stamina.

What yoga has come to mean today broadly consists of several poses called 'asanas' that range from postures to stretching muscles, flexing or extending joints, building core strength, improving balance, increasing our coping ability to challenges, regulating the heart rate, improving breathing, and shedding calories.

Scientific study of yoga does pose some difficulties, though. For one, it remains widely heterogeneous, with as many forms as there are gurus, schools, and practitioners. They come in several names and forms, such as Ashtanga, Anusara, Bikram, Hatha, Hot, Iyengar, Restorative, Vinyasa, Power, and so on. This wide diversity often confuses a novice; whichever teacher he happens to meet first tries to convince him that his form is the best, something akin to what a hotel salesman tries to do to a new tourist who alights at a tourist destination.

The second problem is the challenge of objectively evaluating health outcomes in clear medical terms. While measuring weight, blood pressure, and blood parameters is easy, it is virtually impossible to measure youthfulness, calmness of mind, ability to concentrate, and improved sleep, as other variables such as discipline and diet might also be kicking in.

On balance, yoga seems to have established itself as a credible, important, all-weather, affordable holistic health-promoter-cum-aid for modern-age citizens. It is hardly surprising that it has found wide acceptance in many parts of the world among diverse populations.

Yoga today has two faces: one that is steeped in Indian history and often intertwined with religious philosophy which is promoted by faith-based leaders, prompting followers of other faiths to view it with suspicion.

The other form is a refined, distilled one that has been gleaned by the 'modern' world and seems to be spreading fast. Most practitioners of this form, while acknowledging its roots in India, remain wary of the gurus who have come and gone as fallen angels since the '70s.

Yoga, aptly described by Jigar Gor, is, therefore, "not just about touching toes. It is what you learn on the way. And how you make every cell of the body sing the song of the soul."

08

Shed Weight and Get Fit: Gym or NEAT?

Life is 10% what happens to you, and 90% how you react to it.
– Charles R. Swindoll

Have you ever felt exasperated at the needle not budging despite your fairly regular workouts in the gym? Or is your weight piling up because your painful knees revolt at the thought of running on the treadmill or jogging?

Metabolic scientists have recently discovered that vigorous exercise or workouts in the gym may not be all that effective in burning calories and reducing body fat after all, while NEAT could be the reason why some stay slim and fit without ever visiting a gym.

NEAT is the acronym for Non-Exercise Activity Thermogenesis and refers to that portion of the daily energy expenditure that results from spontaneous physical activity but is not quite undertaken as a part of voluntary exercise.

It turns out that NEAT, meaning keeping oneself active most of the day doing 'non-formal' exercise, could be a great way to burn your fat. Examples include walking up the stairs to your office or home rather than taking the elevator, carrying groceries home by walking rather than using the car, cycling to work, mopping the floor, washing dishes, ironing clothes, cutting vegetables, or doing any or several of the household chores.

That NEAT could be the secret behind many healthy non-gym goers became evident when scientists realised that around 40 per cent of the daily calories are burned by 'just being active' in small ways rather than by the burst of activities in the gym for an hour and then slumping in the chair and ordering others around the rest of the day.

The arithmetic around calories consumed and burned could be depressing. To burn around 120 to 250 kcals that come from eating a stuffed paratha or fried bread requires lifting weights for 30 minutes in a gym.

NEAT helps achieve a more slow-and-steady burning of calories, pushing up the basal metabolic rate for longer periods, thus aiding one to burn more calories, up to an additional 2,000 kcals over the day.

The metabolic disorder package of obesity, diabetes, fatty liver, cholesterol, BP, and increased risk of heart disease is aptly called a lifestyle disorder, where we consume more calories than what we can burn.

NEAT promises to be the way to beat that.

09

Are Artificial Sweeteners Helping You Lose Weight?

Eat for the body you want, not for the body you have. – Anon

If you have been trying to reduce weight by substituting sugar with low-calorie artificial sweeteners and have not lost much, you are not alone. Recent data shows why things may not be working out as we had imagined.

Sugar-containing sweets do cause a rapid rise in blood sugar levels, something that diabetics need to avoid. A wide range of sugar substitutes became available and are now being widely used to add a measure of sweetness to our taste buds. They permitted and perhaps induced us into eating all types of mithai, kheer, pastries, baked foods, soft drinks, candy, puddings, canned foods, jams and jellies, dairy products, and scores of other foods and beverages. Artificial sweeteners had an instant appeal and posed an attractive alternative to sugar because they added virtually no calories to our diet. In addition, one needed only a small pinch compared to the spoonfuls of regular sugar required for the same sweetness.

Many who were trying to shed weight by substituting sugar with artificial sweeteners have been disappointed. Despite the switch to these expensive products, the needle of the weighing machine seemed to have gotten stuck for months. Some were dismayed to see it moving up further right instead.

Doctors at the Mayo Clinic studying this unexpected phenomenon noted that some artificial sweeteners enhanced appetite, thereby making one eat more. There could be a psychological element too, where a person could be eating two pastries instead of one in the belief he is consuming fewer calories overall.

Another explanation is that the brain needs to sense sugar in the blood to turn off hunger. As artificial sweeteners are low in calories, one does not feel satiated easily, thereby making one gorge more along with other diet components, such as starch and fat in a pastry, that could be pushing the weight up.

There are three broad groups of sweeteners in use today. The first group of artificial chemicals include acesulfame potassium (Sunett, Sweet One), aspartame (Equal, Sugar-Free Gold, NutraSweet), neotame, saccharin (Kaltame, Sweet'N Low), and sucralose (Splenda, Sugar-Free Natura). Many of them have an aftertaste, contain no calories, and do not cause tooth decay.

The second group consists of sugar alcohols (polyols) that occur naturally in certain fruits and vegetables but can be manufactured as well. They are not intense sweeteners; they contain some calories (though much less than sugar) and are considered 'healthier'. Examples are erythritol, lactitol, mannitol, sorbitol, and xylitol. They may cause loose stools and could be of help to those with constipation.

The third group consists of natural sweeteners such as date sugar, grape juice concentrate, honey, maple sugar, maple syrup, molasses, and agave nectar. They contain calories, as does refined sugar, and cause tooth decay, but they serve the dual functions of a sweetener and a flavouring agent, especially for some dishes.

Are Artificial Sweeteners Safe?

A recent warning by the World Health Organisation (WHO) against artificial sweeteners has come as a big blow to diabetics and weight-watchers and has set the proverbial cat among the pigeons in the healthcare sector.

Artificial sweeteners had come as a relief a few decades ago for those who were overweight or had diabetes. They were ushered into our foods and onto our dining tables due to steeply mounting health concerns regarding the role of refined sugar whose increasing usage was linked to obesity, type 2 diabetes, fatty liver, and heart disease. Hence they were easily accepted as harmless substitutes.

They have now moved far beyond the cup of coffee and are now incorporated into a range of foods such as cola drinks (especially the 'zero' calorie, 'low' sugar or 'diet' varieties), pastries, sweets, juices, and various packaged products, that we consume regularly.

What is emerging now is that their use could be causing weight gain and metabolic syndrome (diabetes, heart disease, obesity), the very problems they were supposed to prevent. Further, concern is mounting linking some of them with cancer, especially of the bladder.

One of them, Cyclamate, has been banned in the USA.

The possible side effects of artificial sweeteners include digestive disorders, hormonal imbalances, mood swings, increased blood sugar, weight gain, fatty liver, high blood pressure, and an increased risk of cancer.

What could be the mechanisms by which artificial sweeteners harm the body? It is by probably disrupting and altering the normal microbial gut flora, encouraging a new breed of germs to colonise the gut and changing the dynamics and balance of the gut microbiome, thus affecting metabolic well-being.

With the alert issued by the WHO, the use of sweeteners has started to shift from artificial ones to natural ones, such as date sugar, honey, fruit puree, coconut sugar, agave, and jaggery. They are rich in calories, though.

10

Eat Less to Live Long

Mind is the most important part of achieving any fitness goal. Mental change always comes before physical change.
– Matt MacGorry

Restricting the amount of food we consume is a secret tip for living longer. This has been the finding from a recently concluded human trial called CALERIE (Comprehensive Assessment of Long-term Effects of Reducing Intake of Energy) undertaken by the Yale School of Medicine and Pennington Biomedical Research Centre.

The design of the study was simple. Of the two hundred healthy volunteers who participated, some were asked to reduce their intake of calories by around 14 per cent, while others were asked to eat as they normally do, that is until they felt full.

Subjects were evaluated at baseline, one year, and two years for subtle metabolic and immunogenic changes that could suggest effects on life span and health.

Interestingly, those who consumed a calorie-restricted diet showed improvement in their metabolic and immune responses. This was primarily achieved by harnessing PLA2G7, a macrophage-produced protein platelet-activating factor acetylhydrolase that has been established to correlate with healthier lives and longer lifespans.

This study, conducted by two senior scientists, Dr. Eric Ravussin and Dr. Vishwadeep Dixit, went on to find how calorie restriction (CR) was helping the body.

They noted that the thymus gland, located in the upper chest and considered to be the orchestra-master of the body's immune system, showed much less age-related decline in CR subjects; their better-preserved thymus glands could produce more T-lymphocytes that regulate the body's immune system.

Further, CR subjects showed less inflammation in the body. We know that the triad of disordered metabolism, immunity, and inflammation causes ageing and age-related diseases that shorten our life spans. Restricting calories slowed or reversed this process, allowing the body's immune system and tissues to remain young and healthy.

Another aspect of this study was to find out which of the 29 weight-reducing diets was the healthiest. It appears that restricting calories in any form was beneficial; whether it was carbohydrates or fats did not seem to matter much.

The moral of the story seems to be: If you are healthy, get into the habit of reducing your calorie intake. One of the simple ways to achieve this is to stop eating when you are two-thirds full, that is to stop when you still have space in your stomach. Other ways are to skip a meal every day, intermittent fasting, or ritualistic periodic fasting.

Traditional habitants of Blue Zones, the five regions of the world where people usually go on to become centenarians, have several features in common, one of which is following ritualistic fasts.

This could translate into fewer metabolism-related health problems and a longer, healthier life.

11

Foods to Say 'NO' To

Do something today that your future self will thank you for.
– Sean Patrick Flanery

Our health depends on four factors: genes, food, lifestyle, and stress. As there isn't much you can do about the genes that you have inherited, it is best to focus on the other three. What and how we eat, therefore, assumes great importance in shaping our health and lives.

Our relationship with food is paradoxical: it is essential for survival (cliché), but excess of it is emerging as the biggest killer of our times. It pushes us toward obesity, diabetes, hypertension, fatty liver disease, heart disease, stroke, and cancer, accounting for 70 per cent of India's urban ailments and deaths.

Scientists have listed these three foods as the main health hazards of our time:

1. Sugar

These ubiquitous white shiny crystals that were our most common taste-bud tickler and energy booster are emerging as the modern-age 'poison' in these sedentary times, dethroning fats to assume the *numero uno* position. Its consumption has been found to go far beyond our calorie needs. By continuously stimulating the pancreatic beta cells to produce more and more insulin, it tires and knocks them out causing diabetes. Excess sugar gets converted into fat within our bodies, piling up in the liver and causing disease.

Sugar has sweetly sugared its way and entrenched itself on our taste buds and dining tables. Getting rid of it is proving almost impossible. When I asked some of my patients what they offer visiting guests and relatives, they unanimously started their list with cold (cola) drinks, fruit (tetra pack) juices, *nimbu-paani*, tea, or coffee (the syrupy ones that we have grown to love), all laced with sugar, and referred to in health circles as Sugar-Sweetened Beverages or SSB.

2. Fast foods, Fats, and *Trans* fats

Excessive fat consumption is undoubtedly bad for health, but the variety called *trans* fats is among the worst for the heart. Fats are converted into *trans* fats on heating to high temperatures and reheating, as in the subsequent batches of samosas being scooped out of the frying pan or during grilling. They are found in most packaged and precooked foods as well.

3. Packaged and processed foods, food preservatives, and emulsifiers.

These are prime suspects for the surge in obesity, diabetes, heart diseases, and possibly some cancers. The way they interfere with body systems is by disrupting our normal gut flora and replacing it with new ones that make us prone to new-age diseases. Further, their ubiquitous nature and easy availability even in remote regions are causing a major change in the pattern of diseases occurring in cities and towns across many countries.

12

Intermittent Fasting

Diet-wise, I practice intermittent fasting, keeping me alert, as the body is using up its energy stores. It keeps my diet in check.
– Jax Jones

Intermittent fasting (IF) is a form of eating or diet that focuses on timing (a time-restricted diet), in contrast with most other diets that focus on content (calorie-restricted, mediterranean diet, etc.).

The scientific study of IF began with the observation that rodents kept lean by once-a-day feeding were healthier, and lived longer than their counterparts who had access to food throughout the day.

What Does it Do, and How Does it Work?

Ingestion of food stimulates the pancreas to secrete insulin, an anabolic hormone that causes the accumulation and deposition of excess glucose and fat in the liver and muscles as glycogen and fat in the fat cells.

Energy restriction (fasting) for 16 hours or more, results in the depletion of liver glycogen stores and burning of fat from deposits in the body. This occurs as the body in need of energy switches from glucose to fat-based energy extraction, popularly called the metabolic switch. Triglycerides, a type of stored fat, are hydrolysed to free fatty acids (FFAs) in fat cells (adipocytes) and transported to the liver, where they are converted to ketone bodies, acetoacetate, and β-hydroxybutyrate.

Mopping up excess energy arouses the body to undertake maintenance and repair works, improves stress resistance and promotes the recycling of damaged molecules. Fasting stimulates the energy engines of cells called the mitochondria, activates the body and promotes cell survival. All these effects support improvements in health and increase resistance to diseases.

Types of Intermittent Fasting

- 16:8 fasting: In this method, one eats during an 8-hour window and fasts for 16 hours at a stretch. This permits two meals a day while skipping one, either breakfast or dinner.
- Alternate day (AD type) fasting: Complete fasting every alternate day. Water, which has no calories is, however, permitted. This is the toughest IF regime and provides the best results. A less severe form of this regimen allows 25 per cent of the average daily consumption of calories, up to 500 Kcal, on the day of the fast.
- 5:2 intermittent fasting: Fasting for two non-consecutive days each week: One is allowed to take up to 500 calories with black coffee and unrestricted water on the fast days. Normal food (minus refined carbohydrates) is allowed on non-fasting days.

The benefits of IF have been proven by several studies and are as effective as cutting down calorie intake by 30 per cent per meal.

There has to be that moment of fasting, really,
in order to enjoy the feast. – Stephen Hough

The health benefits of IF are weight loss, and improvement in regulation of glucose metabolism (diabetes), blood pressure, heart rate, and cholesterol levels. It has also shown an impressive effect on abdominal fat loss.

The adverse effects are primarily hunger, as the body accustomed to three meals per day since childhood is unable to accept it initially. Those persisting with the regime, however, report declining hunger within a week or two.

A drop in blood sugar levels below normal, or hypoglycaemia can occur, especially in diabetics taking sugar-lowering medications. If their sugars are under tight control with insulin or sulphonylureas, they are advised to try it only under medical supervision.

The concept and benefits of IF seem to resonate with many cultural practices across the world and across time, where faith-based intermittent fasting has been an integral part of traditional life. It offers an explanation for the low prevalence of metabolic disorders, such as obesity, diabetes, and heart disease that we now know are caused by excess consumption of energy-rich foods.

IF offers a simple strategy to harness several metabolic abnormalities resulting from the long-term imbalance between excess calorie consumption and lower expenditure. It could help stem type 2 diabetes mellitus, obesity, fatty liver, hypertension, and coronary heart disease, decrease the chances of getting cancer, and contribute to health and longevity.

13

Remember to Fasten your Seat Belt

Fasten your seat belts. Life does not give you a second chance.
– Margo Channing

The health-related news that shook most of us recently was how the two front-seat passengers escaped death in a high-speed high-end car crash while the two backseat passengers died instantaneously.

This fateful road accident caught much media attention, partly due to the high-profile passenger who died in the crash, Mr. Cyrus Mistry— a young business tycoon and the erstwhile chairman of Tata Sons in his mid-fifties, and partly because the car that crashed was a high-end Mercedes known for its high manufacturing and safety standards.

The question that cropped up was why the two backseat occupants died while the passengers in the front seats, who we intuitively feel should have been more vulnerable, managed to escape. The answer points unequivocally to the single factor: SEAT BELTS!

The front-seat passengers were wearing seat belts, while the backseat passengers were not, and it is being speculated that when a car travelling at a high speed suddenly crashes and comes to a sudden halt, those not wearing seat belts are flung to the front against the front seats, steering wheel, dashboard, or windscreen, as they have nothing to restrain their bodies.

Wearing seat belts for front-seat passengers has been mandatory in India for quite a while now. Thanks to the relentless checking by the traffic police, most drivers and front-seat passengers have come around to accepting the practice. Many of us, however, do not pay much attention or follow seat-belt rules while sitting at the back.

Most developed nations follow strict seat-belt protocols for backseat passengers in their countries. This unfortunate accident has served as a harsh reminder that seat belts are essential for protection, not just for the front-seat passengers, but for backseat passengers too.

There are over 150,000 annual road traffic accident (RTA) fatalities in India, which works out to around 1,200 accidents per day. Research has shown that helmets for two-wheelers and seatbelts for car passengers are the first and main lines of defence, the latter reducing fatality rates by 50 per cent. Airbags are less important and work when the body is restrained by seatbelts.

It is time we learned our lesson from this tragedy and tightened our seatbelts in the back seats too.

Section C

Patient-Doctor Relationship

Without communication there is no relationship.
Without respect there is no love.
And without trust there is no reason to continue.

01

Two-way Patient-doctor Relationship

Patients and doctors need to work together to pursue care that improves health.

Doctors are sometimes accused by disgruntled patients of being unsympathetic, brusque, rude, unprofessional, unscrupulous, money-minded, and many more.

The range of behaviours and attitudes of the patient sitting across the table can be equally varied in spectrum, complexity, and often taxing to the physician.

Indian cities offer the well-to-do patient a wide range of doctors to consult. Hence, with the barriers of fees and waiting time crossed, most patients go on to collect a few or, at times, several opinions.

An anxious young mother had brought her smiling 12-year-old son for abdominal pain and had proudly said that she had consulted 18 doctors, all the very best in town, in the last fortnight alone. Not knowing how best to react, I asked her which of the 18 prescriptions she had tried, to which she said that she had followed none.

A 'second opinion' is a good thing. The situation, however, gets tricky when having collected several prescriptions from several doctors without telling one what the previous had advised, the patient chooses to decide which medicines to take and from which of the prescriptions. This piquant situation often arises when one is not able to trust a single doctor for comprehensive continued guidance.

Many medications can have interactions, and the patient not disclosing the true picture can sometimes land him and the doctor in trouble.

Some patients obviously seem to suffer from an innate inability to trust, but they expect the doctor to go out of his way and take a deep empathetic interest in their welfare.

If a professional opinion is all that is being sought, it is not reasonable for the patient to feel annoyed when the doctor refuses to share his personal number or refuses to take a call in an emergency during off-duty hours.

With the rapidly evolving transactional nature of the doctor-patient relationship, old-world values such as trust, faith, and empathy are beginning to fall by the side.

Politeness, courtesy, professionalism, and appropriate medical care are to be expected from a doctor. No excuses. The problem arises, however, when one starts expecting the additional factors of empathy, kindness, and personal attention to come on as a free add-on, even if they misbehave with the caregivers, just because they have paid the consultation fee.

Patients as well as doctors belong to the human race and have their share of imperfections. Any interaction between them will unfortunately always remain a two-way process.

02

Medical Etiquette

Your degree is just a piece of paper, your education is seen in your behaviour.

Delivering good, gratifying, medical care is very complex as it involves not just knowledge, skills, and ethics, but another component that is often overlooked: medical etiquette.

Medical etiquette is simply good, proper behaviour that is expected of physicians and nurses when dealing with patients.

Simple etiquette is usually not given much importance during medical training in some parts of the world and is often found woefully lacking in several professionals. It is, therefore, not surprising to meet a top-notch specialist with a string of degrees below his name who may forget the etiquette of offering you a seat when you enter his chamber or continue talking on his cell phone while you keep standing wondering what to do.

A resident doctor, who comes to train in a busy hospital, is often grossly deficient in etiquette. In the crowded outpatient department (OPD), I often see him examining a female patient in the presence of several unrelated spectators. In the ward, another common gaffe is barging into the private cabin of a patient without an announcing knock or a *Please, may I come in?*

Poor medical etiquette and poor communication skills are the two most important reasons for patients' dissatisfaction with doctors and hospitals.

Ironically, for most medical colleges (there are over 400 in India now) and hospitals, this topic is not a top priority. As a result, patient visits are often reduced to listening to their symptoms for a few minutes, scribbling a few medications on a prescription pad, ordering a few tests, and scheduling another appointment.

The British introduced the concept of propriety and courtesy in general life as well as in profession. The French word etiquette, while meaning much the same, added a dash of style and grace as well.

Etiquette includes adhering to time, dressing appropriately, being well-mannered, and showing the right measure of kindness and courtesy toward seniors, ladies, colleagues (and enemies too!). It does not come naturally to most and needs fostering.

While etiquette may not decide life and death, what it does decide is whether the patient feels comfortable, cared for, and treated with dignity while in the hospital.

03

How Doctors Think

A man sees in the world what he carries in his heart.
– JW Von Goethe

Doctors may not be the brainiest in society, yet the fascinating ways in which they think and make decisions have been the subject of interesting research. A book by Dr. Jerome Groopman that deals with the subject has hit the best-seller list.

There are some parts of the brain that a doctor uses preferentially over others, memory being the most important to start with. It begins from the time a youngster thinks of taking the entrance test for medical school. He is required to read, retain, and reproduce a large number of facts and names of body parts and functions. Unlike engineering, management, or law students, medical aspirants are hardly required to use mathematical problem-solving, creative thinking, logic, or thinking out of the box. But ask him the names and profiles of thousands of organs, tissues, cells, and drugs, and they will have them at his fingertips!

As they progress to the next phase of clinical work, doctors learn to recognise 'patterns' of symptoms and signs and fit them into the puzzle board of diagnosis. For instance, chest pain accompanied by sweating would suggest a heart attack or jaundice with loss of appetite would fit the pattern of hepatitis.

When the doctor starts maturing as a clinician, he starts to pick up a feature called 'probabilistic thinking', wherein the patient's profile starts becoming a key factor rather than the symptoms alone. To take the example of chest pain again, he starts recognising that the same symptom in a young 20-year-old girl is almost always of neuro-muscular origin and hardly ever from the heart, while in a 50-year-old overweight smoker with high BP, it is very likely to be a heart attack, requiring immediate referral to a cardiac ICU.

With further development in his career, he starts factoring in several aspects of his patient in the process of decision-making. In other words, it is at this stage that he starts arriving at conclusions incorporating text-bookish science that he has crammed. Does the vegetable vendor who has come down with a cough and fever for two days after getting drenched in the rain require to be subjected to a CT scan of the chest, or would an antibiotic suffice? Does the 16-year-old schoolgirl with recent onset vomiting prior to the board exams require an endoscopic examination right away? What if she had had these symptoms last year too, when she was stressed before her final exams?

The mature doctor, then, is not just a repository of facts, information, and knowledge. It is the unconscious assimilation of years of experience, marinated with a sensitive understanding of his patient's concerns and constraints, with a spoonful of intuition thrown in, that makes him take decisions that posterity usually seems to approve of.

Good clinical decision-making, like good wine, matures over time. Knowledge alone does not make a good doctor; wisdom or flavour matters!

04

Second Medical Opinion or Medical Shopping?

In the end, we only regret the chances we didn't take.

When access to medical consultation is as easy and accessible as it is in India, many patients, especially those with resources, do seek more than one expert's opinion.

A second opinion is seeking another medical opinion to verify or validate what the first doctor diagnosed or advised, and it is often quite a valuable step. If an otherwise healthy person who has had no symptoms of disease till yesterday is suddenly told to have liver cirrhosis due to a viral infection that requires long and expensive treatment, it is not unimaginable that he and his family might like to verify the test results, explore if there are other options, weigh the pros and cons, and particularly in our country, see if they can get the treatment at more affordable rates before they decide to start.

The diagnosis of cancer is a common situation as it often comes as a shock and evokes a sense of disbelief and denial in patients, with thoughts like, *It just can't be true; I just had symptoms of indigestion,* or *It cannot be happening to me.* A second evaluation by a competent doctor, reconfirming the diagnosis, helps the patient to accept the unpleasant truth.

Indeed, good physicians and surgeons often advise their patients to consult a second physician to get convinced of the unpleasant diagnosis and then return with greater motivation to embark on a treatment that is expected to be challenging.

It is here that some doctors often fare badly and irresponsibly: Most end up contradicting the previous one, changing the names of medicines in a fresh prescription, and trying to win over and grab the patient rather than sending him back to the first one, sometimes leaving the patient more confused.

The line that divides 'second opinion' from 'medical shopping' is, however, a blurred one.

Medical shopping is quite akin to what we do while buying vegetables: going from one shopkeeper to another, enquiring the rates of cauliflowers, seeing their size, and at times bargaining, before making our purchase. There are people who, in their contrived habit of seeking the cheapest, will enquire about the cost of endoscopy at five centres before going in for one. It may not always be the price, but the popularity of the doctor or the market stature of the clinic.

In most developed countries, medical treatment is somewhat regimented, in the sense that you need to meet your GP first, get referred to a specialist if he feels you need to consult one and meet up with him after you get an appointment. India, in contrast, is an 'unrestricted zone' for medical consultations. Most patients whom I get to see have been to at least four specialists before coming to me.

Once a nouveau riche businessman's wife in her 40s brought her 12-year-old daughter; as I went through her history and scanned the results of the innumerable ultrasound and CT scan tests she had gone through, the mother proudly told me that she had consulted 18 paediatric surgeons and gastroenterologists of the city in a fortnight.

She was obviously in a number game, trying to satisfy herself that she had not left any stone unturned, but was losing out on any doctor willing to take a personal interest in solving the child's problem, knowing he would be just the next one on her unending list.

Medical shopping has its pluses and minuses. On a lighter note, the biggest plus is that it keeps all doctors adequately busy and in business. There is another good side; if most relevant tests have already been done by my predecessors, I find my task of providing an opinion made much easier.

A doctor could have his human frailty too, often feeling he will be yet another number and another piece of paper in the burgeoning file that the patient carries, and find it hard to muster empathy. And it is amusing to see how the shopaholic patient will continue on his or her medical shopping spree, and sometimes come back, as in a game of musical chairs.

Variety and options can be good, but too much choice can often be confusing. In the end, the critical factor is not how many opinions you gathered, but whom you consulted; and then to decide, whom you choose to follow. If the destination is clear and all the paths head that way, then it is up to you to decide how and with whom you wish to undertake the journey.

05

Doctor Gaffes

Laughter is the best medicine.

I am aware that English is not the mother tongue of many doctors around the world. A blend with the local colloquial terms often works well if two-way communication is what matters the most. And with our 'Indianisms', or for that matter the several regional versions of it such as Benglish, Punjish, Tamlish, etc., that we have created so spontaneously, try stopping us from conveying what we wish to, even to the pedigreed English speaker!

It is also an indication of how Indians from diverse backgrounds adapt to a new language. Doctors are no exception to this phenomenon and are as good as others at creating their own phrases and styles.

Despite our lack of proficiency in English, doctors educated in English and practicing in remote regions among people with a mind-boggling range of cultures and dialects, have mastered the art of understanding their patients and communicating with them in strange innovative ways.

So sample and enjoy some of the Doctor Gaffes written on patients' hospital charts or heard during clinical rounds that a prudish lady picked up and posted. Indian doctors would understand what they mean perfectly well, but English speakers might go crazy!

- She has no rigours or shaking chills, but her husband states that she was hot in bed last night.

- The patient has had chest pain when she lies on her left side for over a year.
- On the second day, the knee was better, and on the third day, it disappeared.
- The patient has been depressed since she began seeing me in 2003.
- Past history: The patient has no previous history of suicides.
- Healthy-appearing decrepit 69-year-old male, mentally alert but forgetful.
- Gynaecologist to patient's husband: Between you and me, we ought to be able to get this lady pregnant.
- Occasional, constant, and infrequent headaches.
- The patient has two teenage children but no other abnormalities.
- The patient came out of the ventilator after three days.

You got the meaning in each of them, didn't you? Well, that is, after all, what the role of a language is all about—helping get the right message across, from Indians to other Indians here!

Laughter, as they say, is the best medicine, and we doctors are at your service in providing you with some humour, at our expense this time.

06

A Pinch of Medical Humour

The Art of Medicine is to keep the patient amused while nature cures the disease. – Voltaire

A major challenge that a doctor faces during consultations at times is to keep his face expressionless and straight while listening to the painful stories of his patients. Yes, the stories are almost always painful, as hardly anyone in his normal senses visits a doctor in cheerful good times.

Once, a 50-year-old bearded tall gentleman with luxurious hair and a dense, flowing butterfly moustache came to consult me about the problem of excessive 'gas' in his stomach.

Gas means many things to many people, from bloating, fullness, burping, and belching to flatulence and passing of excess wind down the lower end. After thorough and deep questioning, I concluded that the issue was the last one. While I was scribbling a prescription, he surprised me by saying, "But, doc, farting relieves my distention quite a bit. So please do not give medicines to stop it."

"How do you want me to help you then?" I asked in surprise.

With a troubled look, he pulled his chair closer and said in a hushed tone, "I have come to notice that each time I fart, one hair drops from my moustache." He paused for a while and then went on to voice his real concern, "At this rate, I am worried I will lose my moustache in a couple of years."

Despite many long years of training and understanding that each patient's problem is always unique and requires tailored, individualised treatment, I found my mind groping in the dark for a meaningful response to this rather exotic issue, the like of which I had never heard before. All that I could finally muster up and offer was a prescription of vitamins along with a bouquet of fond wishes and hope that his hair would remain just as dense over the years, and new ones sprout at a frequency that would outstrip the rate of loss due to his frequent farts.

He seemed deeply satisfied, thanked me profusely for understanding his deepest concern, and my offer of help, and made me feel rather inadequate to have to admit that I really had no tangible solution to offer.

As he left the room and the door closed behind him, a giggle that had been building up in my belly for quite a while finally burst through my serious demeanour.

He turned up every couple of months with a fresh picture of his bushy face to have me reassure him that the ebb of deforestation of his moustache had indeed halted.

I soon mastered the art of suppressing a guffaw and donning a serious look each time he visited me. I promised myself a hearty laugh only after I took off the white gown and returned home in the evening.

Section D

Health Risks and Substance Use

The wise warrior avoids the battle. – Sun Tzu

Adult Vaccination

Prevention is better than cure.

The word 'vaccination' has become so synonymous in our minds with the immunisation programme for babies that we forget it plays an important role for ADULTS too.

While we try to ensure each dose for our children, we do not always practice what we preach. Doctors are also partly to blame, as their advice to patients on this aspect is often inconsistent, adding to the confusion.

The table below, taken from Adult Vaccination India, summarises what vaccines we adults need to take ourselves to avoid infections which can be avoided by good vaccines.

VACCINATION SCHEDULED FOR ADULTS					
Age Group (yrs) Vaccine#	Dose	Route	19–49 yrs	50–64 yrs	>64 yrs
Tetanus, Diphtheria, Pertussis (Td/Tdap)	0.5ml	IM	1 dose Td booster every 10 yrs		
			Substitute 1 dose of Tdap for Td		
Human Papillomavirus (HPV)	0.5ml	IM	3 doses (females)		
Measles, Mumps, Rubella (MMR)	0.5ml	SC	1 or 2 doses	1 dose	
Varicella	0.5ml	SC	2 doses (0 & 4–8 weeks)	2 doses (0 & 4-8 weeks)	

Influenza	0.5ml	IM	1 dose annually	1 dose annually
Pneumococcal (polysaccharide)	0.5ml	IM	1–2 doses	1 dose
Hepatitis A	1.0ml	IM	2 doses (0 & 6–12 months, or 0 & 6–18 months)	
Hepatitis B	1.0ml	IM	3 doses (0, 1–2 months & 4–6 months)	
Typhoid	0.5ml	IM	1 dose every 3 years	

A few additional points will help:

- Those who travel a lot or eat out frequently in regions where waterborne infections are common should take the vaccines for typhoid and cholera as well.
- The pneumococcal and meningococcal vaccines are a must for those who do not have a spleen or have weak immunity.
- The varicella vaccine is not required for most who have suffered from chicken pox in childhood. The elderly and those with low immunity are advised to take it. Similar conditions apply for measles, mumps and rubella, and hepatitis A.
- The hepatitis B vaccine (3 doses of 1 ml each at intervals of 2 weeks and 6 months) is a must for everyone.
- The Encephalitis vaccine is useful for adults in areas where this infection is rampant during the rainy season, such as eastern Uttar Pradesh and Bihar.
- And not to forget the COVID shots. We learned about the importance of vaccines from the devastating pandemic of 2020. Ensure to follow the government advisories for new challenges that come along.

Consult your doctor and protect yourself from dangerous bugs lurking around.

02

Enigmatic Vitamin B12

I don't need an inspirational quote. I need a B12 shot.

If you are feeling fatigued, dull, and low, you could well be suffering from low levels of vitamin B12. These symptoms, often passed off as psychological, are increasingly finding their organic basis in vitamin B12 deficiency. Physicians are becoming cautious not to overlook this modern-age deficiency state that can now be diagnosed easily by a simple blood test.

Several problems of nerves and spine, such as tingling of feet, loss of balance, alteration in gait, forgetfulness, drowsiness, and dementia, especially in the elderly, are now being put down to vitamin B12 deficiency, as are fluctuations in mood and even depression. Studies are now showing that it may be the underlying cause of frequent falls and fractures sustained by some senior citizens.

Vitamin B12 plays a crucial role in the normal functioning of the brain and nerves. Also called cobalamin, as it contains the rare element cobalt, and is one of the 8 'B' vitamins essential for most cell functions. Due to its crucial role in the formation of blood, its deficiency slows down the formation of red blood cells, resulting in a low haemoglobin state described as 'megaloblastic' anaemia.

Interestingly, this vitamin is produced largely by the gut bacteria. Equally interesting is the fact that, unlike most other vitamins of the B and C groups that are present in abundance in fresh fruits and green vegetables, this vitamin is present only in animal proteins like meat, fish, milk, and cheese. It is for this reason that vegans, a sect of vegetarians who do not consume animal products in any form, are often found to be B12 deficient despite the body's low requirement of only 2-3 mcg per day.

Symptoms of vitamin B12 deficiency are usually vague and non-specific, often overlapping with other disorders such as hypothyroidism, diabetes, and Alzheimer's disease, making it impossible for doctors to make the diagnosis on clinical grounds alone. Hence, major hospitals and physicians have started prescribing a test for serum vitamin B12 levels in patients with a wide range of symptoms and even in normal individuals coming for a health check.

Some drugs can interfere with vitamin B12 absorption; one common drug is the anti-diabetic medication metformin. Another is the group of acid-suppressant medications called proton pump inhibitors, which have names ending with -zoles, such as omeprazole, pantaprazole, rabeprazole etc... Patients on long-term therapy with these drugs should get their vitamin B12 levels checked periodically.

Once the diagnosis is established, treatment is easy. The vitamin is best replenished by an injection of 100 to 1,000 mcg every 6 to 12 months. Weak and confused patients promptly brighten and spring back to life like freshly watered lilies.

And as I drag myself to work these days, grope for words when I write this book, and scratch my head for the once familiar names, I know it is time for me to take the B12 test.

03

Osteoporosis

Osteoporosis is not an inevitable part of ageing; it is preventable. So it is vital for all of us, of all ages, to start taking care of our bones, now, before it is too late. – Camilla Parker Bowles

A fracture of the hip bone can be the proverbial last straw for an elderly person. We saw a friend's mother go through it all. She used to be petite and frail and had a hump (bent spine). One day she fell in the bathroom, broke her hip, and was bedridden. The orthopaedic surgeon as well as the patient's children, two of whom were doctors, felt scared to subject the 75-year-old to surgery. She, therefore, lay in bed for seven long years, fed and bathed by domestic aids. She suffered the extra misery and humiliation of depending on them for the bedpan as she could not make it to the toilet. Despite all the possible care that the family could provide, she developed bed sores. Her recent death was perceived by many as liberation from her painful, hopeless state.

Each year, there are an estimated 500,000 spinal fractures, 300,000 hip fractures, 200,000 broken wrists, and 300,000 fractures of other bones. About 80 per cent of these fractures occur from relatively minor falls or accidents and are caused by osteoporosis. The stats in India are scary: one in three women above 45 have bones that are fragile; 30 million people are estimated to be suffering from this condition.

Osteoporosis usually has no symptoms and hence goes unrecognised until a bone, usually the hip or the spine, cracks or breaks, often with very minor trauma or a fall. "With every major osteoporosis fracture, the risk of death doubles. Yet it is not taken seriously the world over," says Professor John Allan Eisman, Director of the Bone and Mineral Research Programme, Garvan Institute of Medical Research, and Professor of Medicine at the University of New South Wales, Sydney.

Three factors keep bones strong and healthy: adequate quantities of calcium, vitamin D, and regular exercise.

Calcium, as we all know, is present in fish, milk, and dairy products. For calcium to be absorbed from the gut and deposited in the bones, vitamin D is needed. While adequate exposure to sunshine is considered necessary to ensure abundant supplies of this vitamin, 70 per cent of Indians are ironically found to be deficient in this vitamin despite the hot sun blazing overhead most months.

Recent studies have pointed out that affluent Indians, who can and usually do avoid the sun, are more deficient in vitamin D, while manual workers, who are exposed to sunlight and exercise vigorously, rarely are.

The third factor, and perhaps the most crucial, is exercise. The bones of those who exercise regularly seem to remain thick and strong. Bones, if not put to adequate use, lose their calcium in as little time as a month. This finding explains why hips and legs become weak and fracture-prone in those who do not walk regularly, why women who travel more in cars and walk little, suffer more often from osteoporosis, and why the focus on treatment in the West has moved to regular sessions of dancing or sports for the elderly.

Let us then walk a mile before we sleep.

04

Sunshine Vitamin - the New-Age Immunity Booster

Soak in the sunshine and boost your Vitamin D

Vitamin D, also called the sunshine vitamin, and considered for decades to be needed only for the health of our bones, is emerging as an essential enhancer of our body's immune system. Recent research findings are increasingly ascribing a key immune-boosting role to this vitamin.

Scientists were surprised to find that patients with tuberculosis undergoing treatment with anti-tubercular medicines cleared their infection faster and recovered earlier when given vitamin D in addition.

The research, conducted in England, showed that recovery was almost two weeks faster when vitamin D was prescribed, with the infection clearing in 23 days on average, compared to 36 days if they were given antibiotics alone.

Dr. Adrian Martineau, from Queen Mary University of London, said, "This isn't going to replace antibiotics, but it may be a useful extra weapon, and there could be an even greater role in preventing the disease."

One in three persons has low levels of tuberculosis bacteria in their lungs but has no symptoms, known as latent tuberculosis. However, this turns into full-blown TB in about 10 per cent of them. Prof. Davies's idea is that giving vitamin D supplements, for example in milk, could prevent latent TB from developing.

The idea of using vitamin D to treat tuberculosis (TB) harks back to early times. Before antibiotics were discovered, TB patients were prescribed sunbathing, known as heliotherapy, which increased vitamin D production. Many returned, cured, after a few months of sunbathing in the hills. However, the treatment disappeared when antibiotics proved successful at treating the disease.

Vitamin D is a fat-soluble vitamin that can provide for the body's needs in one of two ways: through the action of sunlight on the skin or through food sources such as cod liver oil, cold-water fish, butter, and egg yolks. When the sun shines on the skin, the ultraviolet rays activate a form of cholesterol that is present in the skin, converting it to vitamin D. Because the body can provide sufficient vitamin D to meet its needs simply through exposure to sunlight, it is called the sunshine vitamin.

Vitamin D is needed to stimulate the absorption of calcium. Vitamin D deficiency causes rickets in children and osteomalacia in adults.

It is now known that vitamin D plays a huge part in boosting the immune system. One of the best ways to prevent colds, flu, cancer, or any chronic disease is with vitamin D. In order to correct the deficiency condition that most people have but don't know they have, 5,000 IU a day is necessary. After taking this much for about a month, you will have filled your need for vitamin D for normal daily requirements.

Many, especially those who tend to forget taking regular or weekly supplements, prefer to take Vitamin D, as an injection: a single shot of 600,000 units. This usually suffices for 3 to 6 months.

It is a pity that we do not use the abundant sunshine adequately and keep ourselves toned, fit, and boosted!

05

Vitamin Overdose

Too much of a good thing can be a bad thing. – William Dudley

Recurrent attacks of severe abdominal pain, renal stones, abnormal moods, and an attack of pancreatitis could well be due to excess consumption of vitamin D. Endocrinologists are seeing patients with abnormally high blood calcium levels due to excess amounts of vitamin D, or hypervitaminosis D, many of who develop serious consequences such as swelling of the pancreas.

A senior nephrologist at our hospital agrees that there is a lurking epidemic of vitamin D overdose resulting in high levels of blood calcium that choke the kidneys and cause renal failure.

Vitamins are catalysts. When taken in very small doses, they regulate the actions of several enzymes and make our body function smoothly. The discovery of this group of substances 100 years ago was indeed a major leap in medicine. Dr. George Wald was awarded the Nobel Prize for discovering vitamin A and proving its crucial role in nurturing the rods in the retina that help us to see by allowing us to perceive light.

The deficiency of vitamins soon came to be recognised, and the dramatic improvement of the patient's condition almost as soon as the therapeutic dose entered the body started appearing as a miracle. Scurvy and delayed wound healing could now be treated with vitamin C; Beriberi with Thiamine (vitamin B1); osteomalacia with vitamin D; night blindness and dry cornea with vitamin A, and so on.

The questions that started being asked were, *Why wait for deficiencies to occur? Why not take extra supplements of vitamins to ensure we don't get deficient in them? If vitamins are 'good' things, then an extra dose should benefit more.*

Unfortunately, that is not always the case. While consuming high doses of vitamins that are soluble in water (vitamins B and C) could be innocuous as the excess amounts pass out through urine, the fat-soluble ones (vitamins A, D, E, and K) on the other hand do not have an easy way out once they get into our bodies. And that is when the problem starts.

The condition of hypervitaminosis D has another angle. With the entry and popularity of bone scans (DEXA scans) and vitamin D estimation tests in India, our scientists reported that as many as 90 per cent of Indians have a deficiency of vitamin D.

What they thought was raising a national alarm in the population's health interests, however, went a bit awry. They failed to define what the 'normal' Indian standard was and shied away from asking that if almost everyone in the population showed a value that was less than that measured in the West, could the 'normal' for us Indians be indeed different?

Vitamin D, therefore, came to be prescribed in higher and higher doses to make bone measurements of Indians meet up with those of their Western counterparts. And while people in Western nations are now reducing their vitamin doses and consumption, Indians are escalating their doses and gulping them down at considerable risk to their health.

06

Tobacco and Today's Health

Tobacco use by humans has had a long and interesting history that is worth reading. Here is a quick recap

The practice seems to date back over 5,000 years in South America. It made an entry into Europe in the 16th century, brought in by the scouts of Cristopher Columbus after he discovered the new world. Jean Nicot, the French ambassador to Lisbon sent a sample to the royal family in France, and thereafter into the rest of Europe. It soon became the most traded item in the world and fuelled the slave trade. It was introduced to the world during colonisation and made its entry into India with the Portuguese.

Tobacco contains nicotine, a name derived from Jean Nicot, and other substances that trigger chemical reactions in nerve endings, heightening alertness and providing pleasure through the release of dopamine and endorphins in the brain.

This mild pleasure soon becomes a habit that evolves into addiction. Long-standing tobacco use is now the single biggest cause of preventable deaths across the world. Tobacco claims lives through a wide range of diseases, such as heart diseases, stroke, lung diseases (chronic bronchitis, COPD), and a range of cancers—lungs, mouth, food pipe, bladder, and pancreas.

Cigarette smoke contains around 5,000 chemicals that are potentially harmful to the body. Its genotoxic (has toxic effects on genes that then lead to cancer) effects are caused by several agents like acrolein, formaldehyde, ethylene oxide, nitrites, isoprene, and acrylonitrile. They induce small changes in the DNA of cells and trigger them to become cancerous.

As regards statistics, there are 1.1 billion tobacco consumers across the world, and one person dies every 6 seconds due to tobacco use. WHO estimates that 5.4 million people died in 2004 due to tobacco and suspects that over 100 million people could have died in the 20th century.

Interestingly, the first report of the harmful effects of tobacco came from Germany in the 1920s, but that voice was drowned in the din of the Second World War. Scientists from the UK drew attention to the hazards of smoking in the 1950s, but global recognition of the dangers of tobacco and concerted efforts to discourage its use started seriously only in the 1970s.

By this time, the tobacco industry had become very large, spread across several countries and had organised itself into a strong lobby to take on the efforts of governments that were attempting to curtail it.

The global and Indian stories, as reported in the GATS 2017 (Global Adult Tobacco Survey) report, do bring a glimmer of hope. They noted a small decrease of 17 per cent in tobacco users and found that nine per cent more people had become aware of the harmful effects of second-hand smoking.

What should we attribute this achievement to? For one, there has been better legislation, large warnings on cigarette packages, banning of *guthka* in several states, and forbidding smoking in public places. The other is increased knowledge or awareness through campaigns and programmes.

What I had learned during my public health fellowship at the University of Sydney, however, still rings. Every smoker knows that the habit is harmful. Why do they still smoke or chew tobacco is an intriguing question.

The answer lies in the first trilogy KAB as explained in the epilogue, where K stands for knowledge, A for attitude, and B for behaviour. Smokers usually have the K but lack A and B which explains their rigid attitude and their inability to stop themselves from the habit they know is bad for their health.

The internal contradiction of the heart digging its stubborn heels to continue the tobacco habit in the face of an avalanche of inputs from the rational mind urging him to stop remains a baffling chapter of human behaviour.

It is not a lack of awareness anymore, as every smoker or *gutka* chewer, from the illiterate labourer to the business baron, is aware that the T-habit harms the body and shortens life. The warning on cigarette packets, especially the foreign-made ones, could not have been louder and more conspicuous. And despite knowing this, millions find themselves either unable or inadequately motivated to kick the habit, putting their own lives and those around them at risk.

India is home to 250 million tobacco users, of which 2,000 people die every day and 900,000 succumb to tobacco-related diseases every year. We hold the first rank in the world with the largest number of patients developing and dying of oral cancer, caused almost entirely by tobacco use. One of our senior political leaders had to be operated on in the USA for cancer of the cheek due to his *gutka-eating* habit. It left its mark by way of a distorted face and an unclear voice that we see every other day on television, as a harsh reminder.

Cigarette smoke contains 43 cancer-causing substances, 15 harmful chemicals, and 400 poisons, all in a single puff. Tobacco contains nicotine, which provides the 'kick' that users enjoy. It is, however, addictive and habit-forming and has zero nutritional or health benefits.

The harmful effects of smoking are well known to even those who smoke: lack of stamina, chronic cough, and increased risk of heart disease, stroke, and stomach ulcers. Smokers are at high risk of cancer, not just of the lungs but also of the mouth, pancreas, and bladder. Contrary to the popular 'macho' image projected by the tobacco industry, smoking reduces potency in men and causes infertility and an increased risk of birth defects in the case of women smokers.

The habit starts at a young age, usually in school or college under peer pressure, often in a spirit of adolescent experimentation or rebellion, and provides that grown-up feeling. The occasional fag then becomes a way of life, a fashion, or personality statement, and then a habit that gets increasingly difficult to kick. The number of smokers in India is growing at an alarming rate of seven per cent annually.

Innocent children and spouses exposed to passive smoking suffer too. They often develop asthma or bronchitis. Sudden infant deaths occur more commonly in homes where someone smokes. Spouses of smokers are at increased risk of developing premature heart disease and cancer. Further, children growing up in a 'smoking home' are more likely to take to it up too.

A T-user is often compelled to stop after the occurrence of a major disease like a heart attack or cancer. But then, one can only look back with remorse that a dash of willpower some years ago could have prevented the irrevocable damage.

Some interesting facts about tobacco: Find out how many you know!

- Currently, over 5.5 trillion cigarettes are produced globally per year. Cigarettes are an attractive and constant source of government revenue because so many people smoke them and are addicted to them.

- Smoking tobacco emerged from religious ceremonies in the Americas and was probably initially restricted to only shamans, priests, and medicine men.
- Ramon Pane, a monk who accompanied Christopher Columbus to the Americas, was first to introduce tobacco to Europe.
- Nicotine is named after Jean Nicot, the French ambassador to Portugal who brought tobacco and smoking to the French court in the mid-sixteenth century as a medicine.
- Anti-cigarette activist and automaker Henry Ford popularised the term, 'The Little White Slaver', referring to the cigarette, in the early twentieth century. Both Henry Ford and Thomas A. Edison objected to cigarettes and refused to hire anyone who smoked, on or off the job.
- Renaissance author Ben Jonson argued that smoking was the 'devil's fart'.
- India ranks highest in the world in oral cancer, caused mainly due to tobacco chewing.
- Two men who appeared in the widely popular Marlboro Man advertisements died of lung cancer, earning Marlboro cigarettes the nickname Cowboy Killer.
- Every cigarette smoked cuts off at least five minutes of life on average, which is roughly the time it takes to smoke one cigarette.
- Within 20 minutes of quitting smoking, a person's blood pressure returns to normal. Within one year, the chance of suffering a heart attack decreases by half.
- Women in the United States increasingly began smoking publicly in the 1920s, when the cigarette was adopted by advertisers as a symbol of equality, rebellion, and women's independence. Currently, cigarette smoking kills an estimated 178,030 women in the United States annually.

- Pregnant women who smoke are more likely to deliver not only low-birth-weight babies but also highly aggressive children.
- A British survey found that nearly 99 per cent of women did not know the link between smoking and cervical cancer.
- The cigarette and cigar are recognised phallic symbols, and several internet sites are devoted to smoking fetishisms. Ironically, smoking has been directly linked to sexual impotence.

The NO TOBACCO DAY comes and goes every 31st of May with awareness campaigns drawing attention to this practice and urging people to discontinue this habit, not just for their own sake but also for the sake of their families and the people around them.

07

Alcohol & Health

Drink never made a man better, but it made many a man think he was better.

Alcohol consumption has played a central role in the social life of people over the centuries. Its entry into the lives of Indians has been relatively recent and has brought with it certain concerns.

- The effects vary significantly from one individual to another; its impact on the mind or behaviour can range from relaxation to sleepiness to euphoria to boisterousness to aggression to violence. It is, therefore, worth keeping in mind that in gatherings and parties, people may behave in unpredictable ways, sometimes ruining the evening with accidents, violence, or aggression.
- It slows down our reflexes, such as in driving, but increases our confidence; hence people are more prone to accidents after drinking.
- Persons taking cholesterol-lowering drugs called statins often experience severe fatigue, muscle pain, and soreness in the body when they take alcohol. This effect is due to both of them (alcohol and statin) competing for the same metabolic pathway in the liver. Medicines that lower triglycerides (fibrates) can sometimes cause severe muscle aches, especially after a drink.

- Certain medicines, including the anti-amoebic drug metronidazole and many others, may interfere with alcohol metabolism and cause severe side effects such as flushing, palpitations, chest pain, or restlessness, a phenomenon described as an Antabuse-like reaction. This is caused by the medication interfering with alcohol metabolism, causing the toxic metabolite acetaldehyde to accumulate in the body. If you are on any medications, check with your doctor whether they are safe to go with drinks.
- The liver is the most common organ damaged by excessive drinking over long periods.
- Pancreatitis is a potentially serious and dangerous complication of alcohol use. Most people who develop it have a long history of significant consumption. It has a unique individual variation—some develop severe abdominal pain with as little as just one drink.
- HOLIDAY HEART SYNDROME. Excess amounts of alcohol consumed during the festive season may cause changes in the heart, from increased heart rate and elevated blood pressure to disorders of heart rhythm. The most common one is called atrial fibrillation, in which the heart beats rapidly and irregularly. It may need hospitalisation, medications, and sometimes an electric shock to the heart to reset the rhythm. It is sometimes associated with an increased risk of stroke and heart attacks.
- Binge drinking, the consumption of excess amounts of alcohol over a short period, typically four drinks over 2 hours, is associated with a higher risk of these complications.
- If you suffer from heartburn or gastro-oesophageal reflux disorder, expect them to get worse with alcohol.

Alcohol is best avoided altogether, but if drink you must, sticking to a single drink for women and two for men should be the upper limit.

Have You Developed a Dependence on Alcohol: Try the CAGE Questionnaire

In our present times of frequent social alcohol drinking, it becomes difficult sometimes to know if one is 'hooked' or dependent. Timely recognition of early symptoms of dependency can help change the course of life.

Alcohol Use Disorder (AUD), as it is presently called, is the wider, all-encompassing term that includes dependency, addiction, and withdrawal, and by virtue of its broad range and blurred margins, it sounds more acceptable as well.

Medical and mind scientists have relied on recognising patterns of behaviour and consumption to identify AUD and have created several scoring methods.

The CAGE questionnaire, an acronym, is one such tool and is the easiest, simplest, and most widely used investigating tool. It consists of four straight questions that need to be answered with a YES or NO.

Here they are:

- Have you ever felt you should **CUT** down on your drinking?
- Have people **ANNOYED** you by criticising your drinking?
- Have you ever felt bad or **GUILTY** about your drinking?
- Have you ever had a drink first thing in the morning to steady your nerves or get rid of a hangover (**EYE- OPENER**)?

Needless to say, the consumer has to answer these questions honestly. The presence of a spouse or relative may help in getting accurate responses to questions 2 and 4.

If any one of the answers is YES, it is time to take heed. It will be good to meet a specialist and seek help to cut down or stop.

After consumption, alcohol is carried by the bloodstream to different organs of the body. It is in the brain that alcohol triggers various moods such as pleasure, desire, relaxation, sleep or anger. The brunt of the injurious effects of alcohol is primarily seen in the liver, pancreas, heart, and muscles.

The effects of alcohol on the brain as well as the body's metabolism and its removal from the body are regulated by a large number of enzymes. The ways and actions of these alcohol dehydrogenase enzymes vary between individuals due to a wide range of polymorphisms or genetic variations.

Hence, we hear stories of someone who drank a whole bottle of whisky every day for decades and did not develop liver disease, while some develop liver damage or pancreatitis with much smaller and infrequent doses; this discrepancy is due to our genetic makeup and how it handles alcohol for us.

Section E

Maladies: Common & Not-So-Common

When you fear something, learn as much about it as you can.
Knowledge conquers fear. – Edmund Burke

I. DIGESTIVE PROBLEMS

Heartburn, Acidity, Lifestyle

Acid reflux: When your dinner decides to ignite a fiery inferno in your chest.

Do you get a burning sensation behind your chest bone, or has sour food come into your mouth? Do you wake up at night with heartburn or acidity and need to drink water or take antacids for relief? If this happens more than once a week, you are suffering from GERD, one of our modern-day maladies.

GERD is caused by the reflux of acid that is normally produced by the stomach into the food pipe or oesophagus due to malfunctioning of the one-way valve located at the stomach-food pipe junction (GE valve). A recent nationwide survey of 25 centres conducted by the Indian Society of Gastroenterology found that 8.4 per cent of Indians suffer from this disorder. If you are a sufferer, you have 80 million people in India for company!

GERD is a lifestyle disorder and hence a phenomenon of our times. Those who are overweight or obese tend to have loose GE valves and are prone to reflux. Alcohol, nicotine (in tobacco), caffeine (in coffee and tea), fatty food (pastries, fried food, cheese, and cream), chocolates, and pungent spices cause relaxation of the GE valve and are notorious for causing GERD, accounting for the early morning heartburn often experienced after that perfect late-night party. An aspirin or painkiller swallowed to clear the headache can worsen the reflux.

The diagnosis of GERD is fortunately not difficult, as the symptoms are quite specific to this disorder. The most common test advised is an endoscopic examination, during which the doctor assesses whether ulcers have formed in the food pipe (oesophagitis) from the refluxing acid chyme. In many patients, with severe symptoms, the changes on endoscopy are surprisingly mild, prompting specialists to coin the term ENRD (endoscopy negative reflux disease). In a few, however, ulcers form in the food pipe, often leading to scarring and narrowing and sometimes to cancer. Lower oesophagal cancer is on the rise in most parts of the world due to the increasing frequency of GERD.

Changes in lifestyle certainly help; the problem today is the practical feasibility of adhering to them. Regular exercises, maintenance of ideal body weight, avoiding all the predisposing foods and beverages, a small early dinner of *sukhi roti* and boiled veggies, and elevating the head end of the bed usually work. Those who can't change their ways prefer to take pills that reduce acid production in the stomach (proton pump inhibitors or PPIs) or tighten the GE valve. They work well, but only as long as you keep taking them. Pharmaceutical companies claim they are safe when taken for as long as 15 –20 years. Longer studies are needed, as many youngsters start in their teens and have 50 years ahead.

Recent research has identified a phenomenon called rebound hyperacidity syndrome in people who have been on PPIs for long periods. On stopping, their stomachs produce large amounts of hydrochloric acid on the rebound, making them dash back for their pills, creating a kind of dependence. Refluxers are often confronted with a life of 'pleasure and pills' or that of a 'frugal pauper'. Not easy!

02

Foods to Avoid If You Suffer from Acid Reflux

In life they are not going to serve you lemons, they are going to serve you lemonade; I really don't like lemonade because I have got a really bad acid reflux. – Felicia Day

Food triggers:

- The most common culprits are oils and fats. Puri and paratha (fried bread) for dinner could give you a sleepless night. For that matter, it could be cheese balls and pizzas as well. Spices, especially the pungent ones, need to be kept away. Malai kofta or butter chicken could make things difficult.
- Citrus fruits or citrus juices are another common culprit. I see several refluxers drinking orange or lemon juice with breakfast and then popping acid-suppressant pills. Non-citrus fruits such as papaya or cucumber are usually fine.
- Chocolate, coffee, and tea often act as triggers. Caffeine loosens the gastro-oesophageal valve, allowing acid to climb up into the food pipe. I have often yielded to the temptation of chocolate after dinner and ended up feeling miserable the rest of the night.
- Fizzy (aerated) drinks are known to predispose. Try watermelon juice instead.

- Alcohol is another common offender. Refluxers learn to identify how alcoholic beverages, especially beer and red wine, make matters worse later in the night.
- Tobacco is a bad perpetrator: It stimulates the stomach to produce more acid, weakens the lower oesophagal valve to let it go up, and further reduces the efficacy of acid-suppressant medicines. It is quite common to see smokers or tobacco chewers not getting relief with the normal doses of acid-blocking drugs.

Life style

- The most important no-no's are late-night dinners and overeating. This is obviously a dampener for partygoers and food lovers. I do not really have any easy remedies for them. A spoonful of Gaviscon (calcium alginate) syrup works well if taken before going to bed.
- Obesity, or let me put it gently, remains a major perpetrator of GER (gastro-oesophageal reflux). It is true that you cannot help solve it quickly, but you need to work on it. I remember a senior defence officer who partied late, ate all that he loved and went to sleep past midnight yet managed to keep his GER in check. The secret of his success was that he went for a 5 km jog every morning, regardless of the weather or the time he went to bed.

  I was filled with admiration but could not emulate him, and preferred to eat less and prudently at dinner instead.

03

Chest Discomfort: Acidity or Heart Attack?

Nothing like a little chest pain to restore your faith.
– Ray Romano

The sudden, untimely death of popular Indian actor Sidharth Shukla in 2021, at the young age of 40, has left many fans and the public shaken and gasping for answers.

He was young and fit and seemed to have been 'fine' and 'normal' until the previous evening.

He experienced chest pain at three in the morning, which he attributed to 'acid' or 'gas'. He drank some water and tried going back to sleep. The pain persisted till the morning, for which his doctor advised him to go to the hospital, but by the time he did, he was dead.

Most 'cardiac' chest pains are no longer as typically described in textbooks: crushing type pain in the centre of the chest, radiating to the left shoulder or arm, associated with sweating or breathlessness.

More often, the initial symptoms are gaseousness, heartburn, or vomiting, and are often put down to indigestion or GER (gastro-oesophageal reflux). Many patients pop antacid pills or drink cold water to soothe their food pipes. Further, symptoms of the two can overlap considerably!

For doctors too, the line dividing "don't worry, take some antacids" or "rush to a hospital right away" pieces of advice is becoming blurred. The traditional differentiators of age, sex, and fitness are not so predictable anymore.

Cardiac deaths are making us redraw our guidelines. They are occurring with increasing frequency in younger people, even in females, and in many who seem to be 'eating right', going regularly to the gym, and maintaining normal body weights. Stress, of course, remains an unmeasurable factor.

The 'heart scare' has already set in. A study revealed that over 50 per cent of those who presented to the emergency room at night with discomfort in the chest had no abnormality on cardiac tests undertaken.

But what about the other 50 per cent? My 35-year-old colleague had visited a hospital at 9 p.m. when a nagging chest pain refused to die down through the day; four hours and two hospitals later, he was diagnosed to have suffered a heart attack. Luckily, he could reach a hospital on time, had an emergency coronary angioplasty, and is hale and hearty six years after undergoing the procedure.

It is good to remember that 'acidity' and 'gas' do not kill, but heart attacks can. The choice is between waking others up at night and going to the emergency room and being embarrassed to be told that the ECG is normal, or waiting till the morning.

Time can sometimes be of utmost importance in matters of the heart.

04

Wheat Intolerance

Being celiac turned my life around for the better. I care about what I eat, I am fit, and my body is in the best shape ever. Crazy that celiac is what opened my eyes.

Many people find it hard to imagine that their intestines could revolt against as innocuous and staple a food as wheat and that it could cause a disease that can even kill. Celiac disease, a condition in which the body reacts to gluten, a protein present in wheat, is well known in the Western world and is on the steep rise in India.

Neha (name changed), a college student from Delhi, came to see me for problems of two to three loose stools every day for four years. Several doctors she had consulted had diagnosed her condition as IBS (Irritable Bowel Syndrome) and prescribed medicines either for infection or to slow her 'hyperactive' bowels. Her relief had, predictably, not been lasting.

What struck me at the outset was her 'thinness'. Although she claimed to eat well, she had a BMI of 17 (normal range is 20–23.5). She also looked anaemic (her haemoglobin was 9). Endoscopic examination of the stomach and large intestine had been normal.

On my suggestion, she got her blood tested for TTG (tissue transglutaminase) and anti-endomysial antibody, which detects wheat allergy, and returned two weeks later with reports that strongly suggested celiac disease. A further test, endoscopy, through which a sample was obtained from the small intestine, confirmed the diagnosis.

Getting this young college girl to stop eating wheat, a staple food and a common ingredient in many items we commonly consume, posed a challenge. Stopping roti, chapatti, paratha, puri, and biscuits for life can be incredibly difficult, especially for people from wheat-eating regions.

For Neha to say no to biscuits, wheat noodles, snacks, and cookies was even more difficult as she stayed in a hostel and did not have many food options. Fortunately, her elder sister, who works as a dietician, understood the importance of the diet regime and offered to cook rice and rice noodles for Neha.

Neha gained three kilos of weight in the next two months, something she had not thought possible for four years. And her energy levels had tripled!

"Celiac disease has already emerged as the most common cause of diarrhoea and weakness in children," says Dr. Ujjal Poddar, Paediatric Gastroenterologist at the Sanjay Gandhi Postgraduate Institute of Medical Sciences, Lucknow. He has worked on this condition for over 15 years. Diagnosing it in adults, 0.8% of whom could be affected with milder manifestations, remains a challenge.

It is quite a familiar entity in the Western world. People with this affliction come together through networks and form their own social groups in cities and regions. A range of gluten-free food items are easily available in departmental stores and grocery stores to cater to their special needs.

While the formidable thing about celiac disease is to stay off gluten-containing food for life, the encouraging fact is that life and growth revert to normal without the requirement of any expensive medications.

Neha has put on another two kilos in the last two months.

05

Lactose Intolerance

My whole family is lactose intolerant and when we take pictures we can't say cheese! – Jay London

Priya (name changed), a 30-year-old office-going woman, came to consult me for bloating, gaseous distention, rumbling in the abdomen, and loose stools for several months. Her weight had been normal. She had undergone several tests, such as an ultrasound, a stool examination, blood work, and a celiac screening, which were negative.

When I asked her if she drank milk, suspecting lactose as a culprit, she denied it, stating that milk did make her uncomfortable and that she had stopped dairy a few years ago. Going deeper into the history, it emerged that her symptoms occurred on days that she attended office, while she remained well when she visited her parents in her hometown. The thought of office stress as a factor did come up in our discussion, but she denied it.

We, therefore, decided that she undertake a simple breath test called the Lactose Hydrogen Breath Test since we were not clear on what was causing her symptoms. A week later, she came back with a report that indicated that she was strongly positive for lactose intolerance

We went back to her history and realised that she had the habit of taking a large cup of coffee (cappuccino) with milk in the office with her friends. On the days she was home and did not take coffee with milk, her stomach behaved well.

The inability to digest lactose, the milk sugar, is emerging as a major cause of bloating, gas, abdominal pain, and loose stools, affecting around 40–60 per cent of adults. Dairy contains lactose, the milk sugar, which needs to be broken down and digested by an enzyme called lactase that our intestinal cells produce.

If the amount of lactase produced by our intestines drops, undigested lactose passes down to the lower intestine, where it is broken down by the bacteria in the gut, releasing gas and irritant products, causing the symptoms.

Lactase deficiency, rare in infants who survive primarily on milk, gets commoner as we grow older. Lactose is present in dairy products, especially milk, cheese, khoya, and several sweets made using them. Curd or yoghurt has very little lactose in it, so people with lactose intolerance can take them without any discomfort.

Avoiding lactose helps manage the situation better, but some prefer to take the enzyme lactase, which now comes as a tablet or drops if they do not wish to give up on their coffee or ice creams.

06

Understanding Constipation

Don't let your poops define you, but they sure feel good when they're successful.

Long-standing nagging constipation may not often be serious, but it acts as a spoiler, detracting from the freshness, fun, and punch of daily life. It is often nagging enough to make the sufferer try out several diets, manoeuvres, home remedies, and laxatives in search of the perfect morning motion.

The first step in assessing a patient with this complaint and understanding his symptoms starts with a few basic questions, as constipation means different things to different people:

- How often do you pass stools? Are they hard?

True constipation is defined as less than 2 (for Indians, 3) bowel movements per week or the passage of very hard stools. By this strict definition, most Indians who complain of constipation may not really be suffering from constipation after all. Their symptoms might mean something else.

- Do you feel a sense of incomplete evacuation after your bowel movement?

For most Indians, this is really the symptom. Bingo! If asked in detail, they will describe their problem as, "I do have movements every day, but I get the feeling that the bowels have not evacuated fully." They often have the urge to go more than once (sometimes several times a day), especially in the mornings, or spend considerable time waiting for a satisfactory evacuation.

If these symptoms are also accompanied by abdominal pain and have been going on for a long time (more than 6 months), they are probably related to a condition called IBS, a common disorder of bowel movement that afflicts one in every ten individuals.

- Do you get the feeling that the stool has come quite low but is stuck near the lowermost end, perhaps requiring the use of a finger or water jet to dislodge and remove it?

If this symptom has been going on for many months or years, it strongly suggests a disorder called 'faecal evacuation disorder', a cousin of the good old IBS. Distinguishing the two can help direct specific attention and therapy to this one.

- Have you noticed blood in your stools?

The presence of blood always indicates the need for special investigation as it heralds a disease: piles or haemorrhoids, which often occur in people who have been straining at stools for years, or anal fissure or crack in the anal region caused by hard stools trying to forcibly make an exit or other causes such as rectal polyps or ulcers.

The most sinister of the causes that need to be looked for and excluded in a person over 40, especially with the recent onset of symptoms, is 'rectal' or colon cancer.

Dietary fibre or stool softeners are a good way to start managing constipation. They also reduce the risk of developing colon cancer if taken for a long time.

But many new medicines are helping to improve the varied symptoms of bowel disorders, adding a dash of comfort and ease to the morning chore and making the experience tolerable, if not enjoyable.

07

Managing Constipation

You know you're an adult when you get excited about a good poop. The secret to a happy life is a good bowel movement!

The symptoms of constipation, IBS, or defecation disorder evoke concerns of the type: What is wrong with my gut? Do I have a narrowing large intestine or an obstruction in my large intestine that is impeding the passage of stools? Could it be colon cancer? Or perhaps an infection, ulcer, or swelling somewhere there?

A thorough history usually helps. One may be able to recognise a temporal pattern with eating late, heavy dinners, consumption of excessive chocolates, caffeinated drinks, and stress (miraculous disappearance of symptoms during vacations or visits to hometown while recurring on resuming office). On the other hand, loss of weight, weakness, joint pain, red eyes, blood in stools, and fatigue could be alarming symptoms.

A good starting point is to ensure that there are no structural or serious underlying causes with a good physical examination, and a few simple tests such as stool examination, especially for occult bleeding, complete blood counts, and sometimes a direct, thorough examination of the large intestine by colonoscopy.

If other variants, such as poor digestion or intolerance to specific foods, are suspected of causing loose stools and flatulence, appropriate tests are indicated, especially for gluten sensitivity and lactose intolerance.

Relief or treatment of constipation hinges on three aspects:

- Getting the character of stools 'just right', that is, neither too hard nor too loose, but with some bulk and shape. Adequate amounts of fibre, as in fruits, greens, and lentils, along with drinking adequate amounts of water help as fibre traps water, swells up, gives form and shape to stools, and keeps the stuff soft.
- The second aspect is ensuring that the evacuation is smooth, satisfying, and all in one go, giving a sense of complete evacuation. This depends on the coordinated contractions of the muscles of the colon. And quite like our moods and behaviours, the muscles of our intestines can choose to be relaxed, coordinated and yielding, tight and difficult, or sometimes sleepy and unresponsive.
- The third is the worrying factor: getting to be sure that all is well down there.

One feature common to most patients visiting a doctor for this ailment is that the medical files they carry when they walk into the consultation chamber are bulky, stuffed with several test reports and doctors' prescriptions collected over the years.

The last four decades have witnessed a huge surge of interest in biomedical research in trying to understand the mechanisms and causes of this common disorder and developing medications and methods to modify bowel movements.

Now there are safe non-absorbable agents such as polyethylene glycol, different types of fibres, and osmotic agents such as lactulose, liquid paraffin, etc., that help soften the stools and give them bulk.

There are now safe medications that relax the major portion of the colon as well as stimulate the rectum by making it contract to expel stools. There are new devices and tools to study colonic motility, along with computerised software to teach the patient how to exert the right pressure at the right places to get that satisfactory motion.

08

Irritable Bowel and Barking Dogs

Life consists not in holding good cards but in playing those you hold well. – Josh Billings

If love is the most misunderstood word in society today, constipation cannot be far behind. A recent study revealed that 5–22 per cent of the population across the world is unhappy with the way their bowels move, and they use the same word to describe a variety of symptoms.

Constipation means different things to different people, from a feeling of incomplete evacuation (45 per cent), straining at stools (30 per cent), hard stools (10 per cent), bloating, and distension (20 per cent), to several others. None of these meet the Western medical definition of constipation, described as the passage of fewer than three stools per week.

How bowel habits differ between peoples and regions, and the urgent need to redefine terms were highlighted during the Asia Pacific Digestive Conference in Kuala Lumpur, in which Asian doctors pointed out that the Western definition of constipation was inappropriate for Asians as hardly anyone would actually qualify while many feel they are constipated while passing stools.

Bowel habits indeed vary widely, not just between people and regions but even between individuals. While many Indians believe that passing at least one stool per day in the morning is crucial to health, it could range from three times a day, often after meals, to once on every alternate day. Timing may not be so important as our modern lifestyle may not often permit us to sit long on the pot before the early rush to school or work, while evenings allow more time to coax stressed bowels to relax and allow passage.

Food and exercise are once again being thrown into centre stage in debates on bowel habits. Our Indian diets of *daal-roti-sabji* have adequate amounts of fibre that absorb water and toxins, give volume to stools, and stimulate the large intestine to move forward with regularity, keeping our constipation as well as our risk of colon cancer at bay. In the USA, bowel cancer has become the most common cancer, making doctors advocate colonoscopic examination for everyone over 45. If we change our food habits to burgers, sausages, ham, and cheese, we will acquire the risks as well, just as Indian immigrants to Western countries have started doing.

A few simple tips can be of use: If stools are hard or infrequent, green veggies and fruits such as papaya, apple, pear, or *bel* (wood apple) can help. If your stool tends to be loose and the frequency is high, try bananas and curd, and cut down on milk and cheese. If gas and bloating are your main symptoms, excess gas-forming foods such as sprouts, dals (lentils), peas, radishes, or milk could be the culprits; try cutting down on them and see if it makes a difference.

Unsatisfactory bowel movements, however, do compete with spouses, bosses, children, and the workplace as a significant cause of unhappiness in life. The solution often lies in treating them as barking street dogs: if you heed them, they bark more; if you ignore them, they often stop barking.

09

Too Much Fibre Can Cause Bloating and Gas

That's what gas is about, that's what the bloating is about and that's what the fat storage is about. – Suzanne Somers

"Consuming fibre in excess of what one's gut can handle is one of the main reasons for excess gas and bloating," said Dr. Kok-Ann Gwee, a senior consultant gastroenterologist from Singapore and President of the Asian Neurogastroenterolgy and Motility Association. He shared his observations of how 86 per cent of rice-eating Singaporeans were troubled by these symptoms when prescribed two spoonfuls of bran, which is considered a healthy dietary supplement in the West.

Indeed, many who decide to turn health freaks and start bingeing on sprouts often end up consulting gastroenterologists for symptoms of bloating and belching.

Milk, in those with lactose intolerance, often causes the same symptoms as undigested food in the intestines, encouraging breakdown by the colonising bacteria and releasing large quantities of CO_2, hydrogen, and methane gases, which stretch the intestines.

Stating that what suits the Western gut may not apply to Asian intestines at all, Dr. Gwee went on to show evidence of how the large intestine of Asians moved two times more quickly than French or Italian ones and how Asians with IBS did not quite fit the Western description of the disease according to the 'Rome Criteria', by being more distressed with the incomplete evacuation of their bowels than with pain.

Researchers from Asian countries have formed a separate group to study and identify the unique features of functional bowel disorders that occur here. Led by Professor Uday C. Ghoshal of the Sanjay Gandhi Postgraduate Institute of Medical Sciences, Indian doctors recently published their observations of 3,000 patients from across the country. Males in India seem to suffer, or at least complain, more than females who predominate in other parts of the world; further, the type described in India is a mixed set of symptoms rather than the constipation and pain variety predominantly seen in Western patients.

The role of diet could be important but not exclusively related to the bowel disorder. Dr. Mahmud Hasan, an eminent researcher from Bangladesh, highlighted the overlap with dyspeptic symptoms in patients with IBS in their predominantly rice-eating population. He also drew attention to the possible role of spices, especially chillies, in both aggravating stomach symptoms, as well as increasing rectal sensitivity, which gives the familiar feeling of incomplete evacuation.

Treating IBS could be as complex as understanding its myriad causes and patterns. In a study described by Dr. Gwee, good dietary advice provided relief in only one-third of patients, whereas most distressed patients required medications in addition. A combination of laxatives and antispasmodics provided relief in half the cases. The best results of up to 80 per cent were achieved when all the components of the syndrome were tackled, often with the addition of acid suppressors and stress alleviators to the cocktail.

Functional bowel disorders (FBD) is a group of disorders where the intestines 'look' normal in appearance and do not show an evidence of anything else that could be serious such as an infection. Despite test reports showing negative results, the symptoms that the patient has refused to go away easily, pointing to a disorder of function (contraction, acid production and so on). They affect around 10 per cent of the population and constitute an ill-understood and poorly managed group of disorders that make many suffer for years. Improved understanding and management strategies are finally helping to bring back the smiles on the faces of these long-sufferers.

Recent progress in understanding FBD shows that disorder of the GUT-BRAIN-axis along with gut microbes could underlie these disorders; hence they have been re-christened DGBI or Disorder of Gut Brain Interaction.

10

Inflammatory Bowel Disease (Crohn's Disease and Ulcerative Colitis)

Your illness does not define you. Your strength and courage does.

The smart, young, 35-year-old, career-oriented Divya's (name changed) problems started two years ago with what appeared to be a usual intestinal infection: cramping abdominal pain, loose stools, and feverishness. She took her regular antibiotics, and although the symptoms improved slightly, they lingered and persisted.

Over the next six months, she had four major bouts, lost 6 kg of weight, became anaemic and weak, and passed blood in her stools a few times. She finally consulted a gastroenterologist who performed a colonoscopy, a test which requires passing a flexible tube through which one gets to look into the large intestines and diagnosed her to be suffering from Crohn's disease.

Like most people her age, she had never heard of Crohn's disease. It is an autoimmune condition in which the body's immune cells, normally primed to target and kill invading germs, get misdirected and start attacking the intestinal cells of its own body.

Her husband, a TV channel manager, was shocked too. The questions that seemed to flow endlessly in their minds were: How did it happen? Why did it happen? What is the cure? How long will it take? Will it impact her career? What about their plans for a baby?

To be rudely woken up into the world of inflammatory bowel disease, the generic name for Crohn's disease and ulcerative colitis, cannot obviously be pleasant.

Most answers initially appear to be negative: the exact cause is not known, the disease does not have cure, and sometimes requires surgery.

How long should I take the medicines?

Lifelong!

Are you serious? And can it turn cancerous?

Yes (it may, after many years).

OMG.

Divya, who is now well and back on her job, needs to take some tablets regularly. She will tell you how bad it could get. Initial disbelief led to anger and then to frustration. It was several months later, after several consultations, opinions, and reading up on the net, that she and her husband finally accepted the reality and decided to fight on.

Thanks to a new group of medicines called 'biologicals', she got well quickly, gained weight and started feeling normal again.

Steroids, once the mainstay of therapy, are now prescribed reluctantly due to their long-term side effects. Remissions are easy to achieve, and one can expect to lead a near-normal life.

IBD or Inflammatory Bowel Disease as they are called, are of two types: Ulcerative Colitis, the commoner one where ulcers develop in the colon or large bowel, and usually come to attention due to persistent frequent loose stools, often with blood, and the other called CROHN's disease, that Divya had.

There are six levels of treatment, the choice depends much on the severity and extent of the disease, as well as the preference of the doctor and patient.

Biologicals are costly. Luckily, Divya had health insurance to cover the costs for a while.

The mildest therapy is a group called amino-salicylates, moving up to steroids, immune-modulators, biologicals and so on. More affordable alternatives called 'small molecules' (such as Tofacitinib, Etrasomod and their likes) are now hitting the market, some proving to be almost as effective as biologicals. They are brightening up the prospects of patients suffering from IBD and are most promising in times to come.

Every organisation has some staff who suffer from this group of conditions. It is time we unite and create awareness about this disease so that anyone afflicted does not have to suffer in isolation or shame. And we can bring help and information to their doors.

11

Gallbladder Stones

It is better to be unhappy and know the worst than to be happy in a fool's paradise. – Fyodor Dostoyevsky

"Lazy good-for-nothing stoner! RIP gall bladder."

Once, a young lady from a group of young visitors to our hospital volunteered to lie on the couch to have me demonstrate how an ultrasound machine works. When I put the probe on her abdomen, intending to show them what normal organs in the abdomen looked like, I was surprised to find that her gallbladder was packed with multiple stones. On repeated questioning, she denied having had pain ever.

It is very common to form stones in the gallbladder. Of every hundred adults walking on the streets in northern India, stones will show up in the gallbladder in at least five of them if they are all subjected to an ultrasound test. This figure goes up to around 15 in Western Europe and America. The highest prevalence of gallstones has been reported in a tribe of Pima Indians (native Americans), 75 per cent of whom are affected by the age of 35.

Why are stones formed in the gallbladder of some individuals is still not clear. Medical students are often taught the risks of the six Fs: fat, females, forty, fair, fertile, and those with a family history. Though females are more often afflicted than their male counterparts, and fatty people indeed more often have stones, they need not have to be fair anymore to qualify for having them.

Gallstones usually appear yellowish or whitish and are composed of cholesterol. They form due to excess amounts of this sludgy material that the liver excretes in the bile. Around 15 per cent of stones, however, are black in colour and consist of a black pigment formed from the breakdown of bilirubin.

Medical scientists distinguish two types of stones: the naughty ones that come to attention by causing severe pain and the silent ones that are picked up incidentally. The painful ones are likely to cause pain repeatedly and are best removed by surgery.

Doctors seem divided in their opinions about how to deal with silent gallstones. Dr. Gracie followed up with a group of 200 Americans with silent stones for several years in the 1980s and found that only 18 per cent developed pain in their lifetime. In other words, 82 per cent went through life harbouring stones without any problems. The conservative group, therefore, feels that silent stones are best left alone unless they start giving trouble.

The aggressive group, on the other hand, is composed mainly of itchy-handed surgeons who recommend that stones are best removed before they cause trouble. They point to rates of potentially serious complications such as pancreatitis (1 per cent) and cancer (0.6 per cent) and argue that the benefits of laparoscopic surgery in modern times far outweigh its risks. Why live with the constant worry that the stone may slip one day or the gallbladder may turn cancerous?

A senior lady doctor who had sought my consultation for silent gallstones a few years ago finally underwent surgery and got her gallbladder with stones removed. "I don't have to worry about them every day anymore," she told me when she met me at a party.

II. PROBLEMS OF HEART

Look after your body. That is the only place you have to live.
– Jon Rohn

Chest Pain

I got a heart full of pain, a head full of stress, handful of anger, held in my chest. – Linkin Park

Pain in the chest is indeed common in the Indian community, with around one in four people suffering from it at some point in their lives. The pain in this part of the body has a peculiar, sinister undertone, suggesting that it could be arising from the heart and ushering a threat that it might kill.

In fact, the medical word for chest pain that arises from the heart, 'angina', literally means 'impending feeling of death'. In its classical form, it is described as a feeling of heaviness or crushing pain in the centre of the chest that sometimes radiates to the left shoulder, back, or neck. Typically, it is brought about by exertion, such as during a brisk walk, and often abates within a few minutes of pausing.

For much of my career, I used to think that cardiac chest pain occurred only in men above 40 years, especially if they smoked or had associated conditions such as obesity, diabetes, high blood pressure, increased cholesterol levels in the blood, or family history.

This profiling does not seem very reliable these days, as I have been proven wrong on quite a few occasions. The most startling case was the young wife of my office typist, who casually walked into my office with a smile one morning to seek some medicine for frequent attacks of chest pain, which I suspected to be due to acidity.

The next morning, I saw loud conversations in the corridor. As this girl's chest pain persisted, she was brought to the emergency at night, when an abnormal ECG led to an emergency angiography. One of her coronary arteries was found blocked and an angioplasty had to be done at the same session to restore blood flow to her aching heart muscles. She walked out the next day, free of chest pain.

Fortunately, two-thirds of patients with chest pain presenting to the emergency, turn up to have normal heart tests. This has led to a new term called NCCP (Non-Cardiac Chest Pain).

In most instances, the pain arises from the food pipe or oesophagus. This muscular tube often goes into spasm when acid from the stomach refluxes into it. Gastro-oesophageal reflux disease or GERD as it is called, is indeed so common that doctors recommend a simple 'acid suppression test' with a double dose of acid suppressants for a few weeks to see if the pain settles and so does the concern.

Nagging chest pain can have its origins in other organs too, such as the lungs, muscles, nerves, and bones. Swelling and inflammation of the ribs, called costochondritis, can be particularly painful and disabling.

What remains at the heart of the issue is to exclude the heart as the cause of pain. And with heart disease occurring more commonly in young people these days due to changing demographics and lifestyles, distinguishing non-cardiac from cardiac chest pain is getting more challenging by the day.

02

Young Hearts are Under Attack

Life never gives us what we want at the moment that we consider appropriate. Adventures do occur, but not punctually.
– EM Forster.

What has caused considerable concern among cardiologists in recent years is the observation that young, apparently healthy men in their 30s and 40s are becoming victims of heart disease. Once considered a malady of the elderly, it is emerging as a major health problem among young Indians.

When Shailender, a cheerful 41-year-old clerk of our department, complained of gas and heaviness in the upper abdomen one morning two years ago, he was prescribed the customary digene tablets. When he insisted on showing the cardiologist, his colleagues called him a hypochondriac. A day later, we were startled to hear that he had to undergo emergency angiography and stenting the previous evening for an acute myocardial infarction.

There are nine conventional risk factors for heart disease that cardiologists talk about—obesity, diabetes, smoking, high blood pressure, alcohol, lack of physical exercise, abnormal blood lipids, a strong family history of heart disease, and stress. The interesting fact is that the risk increases from two-fold for one risk factor to 300-fold for all nine, implying that as risk factors get added, the actual risk literally multiplies. The optimist would, however, realise that except for family history, all the other risks could be controlled with lifestyle changes or medicines.

There was, however, no obvious risk in Shailender's case. He looked and weighed normal (his BMI was 23), had normal blood pressure, was a vegetarian, and did not have diabetes. Like many, he had been a smoker for five years but had quit since marriage. His blood lipids were normal. Then, why did he have a heart problem?

The rather common occurrence these days of heart disease in young people without any of the conventional risks is challenging this neat theory of 40 years. The country was shocked a few months ago by the sudden death of one of the youngest CEOs and health freaks, Mr. Ranjan Das, at 42 in Mumbai. He ate right, was a marathon runner, had regular executive health checkups, and was considered a model of perfect health in the corporate world.

Indian cardiologists admit that the frequency of heart disease in India is one of the highest in the world; further, it occurs around 10 years earlier, is more often fatal at first presentation, and tends to be more severe (where all three coronary arteries are affected).

Three theories are doing the rounds. Some pundits are driving down the upper limits of lipids, claiming that levels of cholesterol and triglyceride exceeding 150 and 160 could damage Indian hearts. Also, an LDL-Cholesterol level of more than 70, an HDL-Cholesterol level of less than 40, or an increase in apolipoprotein A could be damaging.

Physicians who are more pragmatic have started to look beyond. Stress and sleep deprivation are emerging as major contributors. A lack of reliable methods for quantifying them poses major hurdles to scientific research. Seven hours of sleep every night might help the stress-related body revert to normal and protect our hearts. It is time we got ourselves more sleep.

03

Can Heart Attacks Be Induced by Stress?

We need to stop glamorising overworking. Too many people wear their burnout as a badge of honour. – Katy Leeson

The sudden death of 53-year-old Indian singer KK of a heart attack after a gruelling evening performance in an overcrowded hall has shocked not just the public but medical scientists too.

The circumstances do not seem to leave much room for doubt. He was a non-smoker and was not known to suffer from the usual risk factors such as diabetes, hypertension, obesity, high cholesterol, or previously known heart conditions. Many who knew him personally, testified on television that he was quite a health freak with no bad habits.

What then could have caused this sudden fatal heart attack? Circumstances clearly suggested stress, that nebulous factor which scientists have not yet learned to define and measure. 7,000 people were thronging an auditorium meant for 2,500; it was unusually hot in there due to lack of adequate air-conditioning. The show required him to sing 20 songs back-to-back, perhaps as a part of the contract. And to top it all, he had to put on a friendly, high-energy appearance to keep the audience entertained despite being uncomfortable and sweating.

Medical science often tends to deny the existence of 'stress', something that it finds difficult to prove or measure, although it may look fairly evident to the common on-looker. Let me, therefore, share another episode from recent times.

Joe Garcia, the 47-year-old husband of one of the two teachers slain along with 19 children in the devastating school shootout at Uvalde, Texas, died of a heart attack the next morning. The circumstances compel us to invoke that nebulous trigger again: it was not just the loss of his wife of over 24 years, but the agony and unexpected manner in which it all happened.

He died suddenly, soon after attending the memorial service of his wife, from what the press described aptly as 'a broken heart'.

Observations strongly indicate that unusual stress, whether physical, mental, or emotional, can precede or induce a heart attack; and cardiac events are the most common cause of death across the world, particularly in urban India.

Learning how to manage stress may not sound all that scientifically erudite, but awareness, insight, and preventive strategies to cope and deal with may hold the key to our survival when conventional medical knowledge has not caught up quite yet.

04

Cardiac Arrest: Lessons from the Football Field

A heart can stop beating for a while, one can still live.
– Suzanne Finnamore

The term 'Heart attack' implies that the arteries carrying blood to the heart muscles are narrowed or blocked, causing pain in the chest and damage to the muscles.

What happened to Christian Erikson, the 31-year-old midfielder of the Danish team, on the football field in 2021 was somewhat different. He collapsed suddenly during a match when his teammates realised that his heart had stopped beating. They could not feel his pulse. He had suffered a cardiac arrest, a state in which the electrical activity of the heart, which causes the muscles to contract, had ceased.

This episode, widely watched all over the world on television, has come as a huge lesson to most. Erikson's teammates, who were the first to attend to their collapsed colleague, quickly got over the initial shock, cleared his airway, put him in an appropriate position, started the cardiac massage and called the paramedics.

Erikson received external cardiac massage (CPR for cardio-pulmonary resuscitation), a special way of thumping and pressing the chest to try and restart a stopped heart. An electric shock was then applied to the heart using a defibrillator (AED: automated external defibrillator). By the time he was carried off the field, his heart had resumed beating, and he had regained consciousness.

Erikson was monitored in a hospital for two days and then discharged. Since his heart runs the risk of stopping again, he was advised to have an ICD (intra-cardiac defibrillator device) inserted in the future.

Contrary to popular belief, cardiac arrests occur in young and fit people too. It can occur to any of us.

What would you do if someone at home collapsed in a similar way? Call the doctor? Or ambulance? If blood supply to the brain or heart muscles stops for more than five minutes, the organs are damaged beyond repair.

The only hope for restarting stopped hearts and reviving people back to life is if someone there or nearby who knows how to perform cardio-pulmonary resuscitation or CPR, and if by the time an ambulance arrives, they can switch to an automatic external defibrillator (AED).

All these tips and methods are packed into an essential course called BCLS (basic cardiac life support); every medic, nurse, ambulance driver, teacher, physical instructor, school principal, and for that matter, EVERYBODY needs to know. It might be possible for you to save a life through timely intervention.

In Europe and England, there has been a 2,000 per cent increase in visits to websites and applications for training in BCLS. It is time to wake up and learn the basic steps of what to do in an emergency.

01

III. LIVER PROBLEMS

Fatty Liver Disease: Emerging Therapies

Is life worth living? It all depends on the liver. – William James

Fatty liver does not only occur in alcohol conusmers. Non Alcoholic Fatty Liver Disease (NAFLD), that has recently been rechristened MASLD (Metabolic Dysfunction Associated Steatotic Liver Disease) has emerged from an incidental, inconsequential disorder to a major cause of early deaths, not just from liver failure and cancer, but more often from cardiovascular diseases.

Insulin resistance appears to be the underlying mechanism that sets the damage sequence of this condition in motion. Hence, the treatment of MASLD has revolved primarily around weight reduction strategies, be it through lifestyle alterations such as weight-reducing diets and exercise, or bariatric procedures such as gastric balloon insertions or bariatric surgery.

Understanding MASLD at the molecular level has led to the development of new compounds that target specific steps in the pathogenetic or damage-sequence pathways of this condition. These include agonists or stimulants of PPAR (peroxisome proliferator-activated receptors) such as Saroglitazar.

This molecule developed by an Indian pharmaceutical and has become the preferred treatment by most liver specialists due to its safety and effectiveness.

Several other medicines designed for treating type 2 diabetes, are gaining ground rapidly. One group called the SGL2 Inhibitors and taken orally (empagliflozin and dapagliflozine being common names) are being preferred by diabetologists for obese diabetics with fatty liver. They squeeze the extra fat out from the liver and bring down the sugar as well.

Another group of medicines that is hitting headlines is called GLP1 agonists (common names: semaglutide, liraglutide); they are effective for all three: diabetes, fatty liver and weight reduction. Earlier available as weekly injections Semaglutide is now available as a tablet. Its brand name (Ozempic) got a mention at the Oscars recently, as it is effective for weight reduction that celebs often seek.

02

Fatty Liver and the Heart

A liver stuffed with fat takes its revenge on the heart.
– Gourdas Choudhuri

Fatty Liver, which commonly is mentioned in an ultrasound examination report and is often passed off as an incidental finding, may not be innocuous after all. Japanese and European scientists have noted a four-fold increase in the risk of heart disease in patients with fatty liver compared to those of the same age and sex with lean 'normal' liver.

Using sophisticated techniques, doctors have found the walls of arteries to be thicker and their lumen narrower in patients with fatty liver, resulting in reduced blood flow to the heart muscles. Their findings explain why those with excess fat in their livers are more vulnerable to dying from heart problems.

The appearance of a 'bright' and swollen liver, indicating surplus fat, is a common finding on ultrasound examination. It used to be commonly seen in heavy drinkers but is nowadays often seen in teetotallers too. Hence the new name non-alcoholic fatty liver disease or MASLD. Although the risk of liver damage due to this fat is modest and occurs in only 20 per cent of people when present for over 20 years, the chances of heart attacks are grossly increased.

MASLD is usually seen in individuals who are obese, have diabetes, or hypertension, or suffer from high amounts of circulating fats in the blood. This constellation is called 'lifestyle disorders' and they make up what is medically called metabolic syndrome. Lack of adequate exercise and consumption of excess calories are often the two main culprits that lead to obesity and excess deposits of fats.

The mechanisms underlying this disorder, called Insulin Resistance, are similar to that which occurs in diabetics of the type 2 variety or the common adult type, in which patients have high circulating levels of insulin that prove ineffective in driving sugar into cells. Insulin Resistance also causes excess accumulation of fat in liver cells as well as thickening of arteries that cause heart or brain disease.

Regular exercise and reduction of weight form the fulcrum of treatment for this disorder. Apart from helping reduce weight, aerobic exercise activates a protein (glut-4), that restores the sensitivity of cells to circulating insulin. Hence insulin and sugar levels both come down, fat gets mobilised from the liver, buttocks, and abdomen, and the risk of heart disease is back to normal levels.

India is the epicentre of a global epidemic of diabetes and heart disease. While our genes may be partly accountable for our misfortune, the greater share of blame lies in our reluctance to exercise regularly. The vagaries of weather and unsafe roads notwithstanding, we, more than any other race, need to shake off our laziness and indulge ourselves in far more regular exercise than what we are doing at present. And we need to start quite urgently if we want to live longer and healthier lives.

03

Food Fads in Liver Disorders

My biggest regret is putting my body through fad diets.
– Jennie Garth

In an attempt to do well for those they love, spouses and parents often enforce diets on patients with liver diseases that often turn out to be detrimental.

Most commonly, pale food and insipid boiled cabbage are doled out to nauseous patients suffering from hepatitis, which makes them puke even more.

The liver, in a way, is a buzzing manufacturing unit that requires lots of energy to keep its multiple functions going. And it derives it from the food we eat.

During an attack of jaundice, when many of the liver cells are injured or killed, the liver attempts to recover by regenerating its cells quickly. For it to happen, it requires a generous supply of energy that comes from carbohydrates and proteins, the building blocks of tissues.

Boiled green vegetables, unfortunately, have neither of these. Hence, the situation often progresses to that of a starved liver unable to recuperate due to a cut-off in food supply.

Recent studies are beginning to show how an adequate supply of energy and protein through nutritious food during this critical phase revives damaged livers. Carbohydrates (starch and sugar), the most important sources of energy, are sourced from rice, sugar, idlis, idiappams, sooji, and noodles, as are fruit juices and sweets such as rasgullas, which need to be given liberally.

Interestingly, fat, thought to be toxic to livers, is not prohibited if taken in moderation. Each gram of fat provides nine kilo-calories, compared with only four that come from carbohydrates. That patients do not enjoy fried food at this stage of their illness is, of course, another matter.

Adequate importance has not been given to protein, the other important ingredient our livers need most. International guidelines recommend a diet of 1 to 1.5g per kg of body weight per day to meet the liver's increased requirements. Here again, the spotlight has shifted from conventional animal sources (meat, chicken, fish, eggs, milk, curd, and cheese) to those derived from vegetarian ones such as dals, rajma, and soya.

Soya is perhaps the most useful and yet the most neglected item. It is not only rich in protein (40 per cent) but also contains a large proportion of branched-chain amino acids (BCAA) that are specifically beneficial in liver disease. Eating soya chunks at least once with lunch or dinner can do the liver much good.

Last but not least unreasonable practice is withholding *haldi* or turmeric from cooking. This stems from associating its yellow colour with that of bilirubin, the compound that gives jaundice its yellow hue. The link is as stupid as feeding tomatoes, which derive their red colour from a pigment called anthocyanin to anaemic patients with low haemoglobin levels. We need to look beyond colour.

Patients' relatives often expect doctors to write merely medicines in their prescriptions, taking upon themselves the decision of how to feed ailing relatives. No harm. As long as we update ourselves and rid our minds of senseless fads.

04

Hepatitis

Jealousy is the jaundice of the soul. – John Dryden

Q1: What does the term 'hepatitis' mean? When do you diagnose it?

Answer: Hepatitis means diffuse injury to the liver (hepar means liver, itis means inflammation) in which hepatocytes or liver cells die at a fast rate. When this happens, the cells release enzymes such as SGOT (AST) and SGPT (ALT) into the bloodstream, which accounts for the abnormality seen in liver function tests.

Q2: What are the types of hepatitis?

Answer: There are two broad types: **Acute** hepatitis refers to an illness that has occurred in a short time. It is characterised by a marked increment in the level of liver enzymes, usually in the thousands (normal levels are usually around 40 IU/L). The other is **chronic** hepatitis, in which liver damage occurs indolently over more than six months. Liver enzymes may be mildly increased, or sometimes even normal, in this form.

Q3: What are the common causes of acute hepatitis? What is the danger?

Answer: The most common causes are infections of the liver due to viruses A, E, B, and C (hepatitis A, hepatitis E, hepatitis B, and hepatitis C). Sometimes, the liver could be reacting to certain medicines or chemicals. It is often associated with nausea, loss of appetite, pain in the tummy, jaundice, and yellow urine.

Most patients (more than 95 per cent) with hepatitis A and E usually recover over four to six weeks, as the body fights out and gets rid of the virus and regenerates the liver. Rarely, the liver fails pushing the person into a liver coma.

Q4: What causes chronic hepatitis, and what could be the consequences?

Answer: Slow damage to the liver can be caused by certain infections such as hepatitis B or hepatitis C, regular high alcohol consumption, and excess deposition of fat in the liver (fatty liver). Rarer causes include autoimmune hepatitis and metabolic disorders such as Wilson's disease and hemochromatosis.

Although the degree of liver function abnormality is not that dramatic in this form, chronic hepatitis often leads to a condition of scarring and weakness of the liver called liver cirrhosis. The risk of developing cancer of the liver also goes up in patients with chronic liver disease.

Q5: How does one get to know if he has a weak liver?

Answer: Acute hepatitis is diagnosed by clinical symptoms, elevated liver enzymes in blood tests, and further, by tests to detect which virus (A, E, or B) is causing it. Another blood test, called prothrombin time, tells us if the liver is in danger of failing.

Chronic hepatitis may not be detectable clinically and requires tests for diagnosis. Blood tests for liver functions (liver function test or LFT), hepatitis B (HBsAg), hepatitis C (Anti-HCV), and a fibroscan test help tell if there is anything to worry about. If all three are normal, you have a healthy liver.

Q6: Is it necessary to do all these tests on a person who feels quite normal?

Answer: It is certainly desirable, as detecting and treating a liver disease at an early stage prevents the development of liver cirrhosis. Very effective treatment is now available for hepatitis B and hepatitis C and early stages of chronic hepatitis can be reversed completely.

When symptoms of liver cirrhosis such as swelling of the feet, water in the abdomen, bleeding in the intestines, and weakness develop, it becomes difficult to restore the liver to normal. One may then have to undergo an operation called liver transplantation to restore a healthy liver.

It now takes only five minutes to detect early liver damage with a simple, painless test called liver fibroscan. Early detection pays huge dividends by ensuring that your liver recovers and remains healthy for life.

Hepatitis B

When Siddharth (name changed), a 22-year-old, went to donate blood for his mother's treatment, he was shocked to hear that he harboured a hepatitis B infection. He was fit, played for his college cricket team, and had not suffered from jaundice which explained his disbelief.

Hepatitis B is usually a silent infection. One of the global awareness campaigns *Am I Number 12?* was aimed at drawing attention to this frequency. In India, the rate is somewhat lower; 43 of 2,500 apparently healthy people tested positive during a free checkup camp in the city. Around 20–40 million people in India are infected with hepatitis, six to ten times more than HIV. It spreads through infected reused needles, poorly tested transfused blood, the sharing of instruments such as shaving blades or ear-piercing needles, from a carrier mother during childbirth, or unprotected sex with an infected person.

What makes hepatitis B worrisome is it is silent for many years, during which the virus nibbles away the liver cells, ultimately leading to liver failure (cirrhosis) or liver cancer. These individuals have felt quite normal for years. When symptoms do appear, much of their liver is already badly damaged.

Siddharth was lucky to be diagnosed before his liver was severely damaged; he was put on medications with which the infection was now well suppressed. His mother, who had vomited blood, was diagnosed with cirrhosis from a prolonged infection with the virus. His younger brother also tested positive, both children having probably acquired it from her during childbirth.

A screening test for hepatitis B has become a standard recommendation during antenatal checkups so that the newborn of a carrier mother can be protected with immediate vaccination and hepatitis B immunoglobulin injections just after birth. It is hardly followed, as facilities for testing are not available in most government hospitals, community centres, and primary health centres. Routine vaccination of newborns with the vaccine (costing Rs 8 per paediatric shot; three shots are required for full protection, a month and six months after the first shot) has still not been included in the government vaccination schedule in most parts of India. More than 150 countries, some less economically developed than ours, have adopted it and brought down the infection rates drastically.

The vaccine used to be fairly expensive, costing Rs. 1,500 for three adult doses. With many companies manufacturing it, the cost for three doses has dived to around Rs. 50 for a lifetime of protection. Despite this, we found that only one-third of school students in Lucknow had received the shots. The rates were as low as zero per cent to six per cent in rural schools. The issue is less about cost and more about awareness. While Gates and other foundations have helped spread awareness about HIV infection, hepatitis B, which infects and kills more than ten times as many people as HIV, is at large.

Hepatitis C

Hepatitis C, a small RNA virus that causes infection and damage to the liver, had its moment of public recognition when the well-known silver screen celebrity Pamela Anderson of Baywatch fame was diagnosed with it. The way she contracted it was equally sensational: She had shared the needle for a skin tattoo with her boyfriend, Tommy Lee, who carried the infection. The gossipy tale went further, with her litigating against him for concealing the information, but as often happens there, they finally united in wedlock.

Hepatitis C infection is indeed more common than most of us probably know. Of all of us who consider ourselves perfectly healthy and volunteer to donate blood, one per cent harbour the infection. In other words, approximately ten million people in India have the infection and do not know it.

The hepatitis C virus is a stealthy one that hardly ever produces jaundice, the commonly known symptom of liver disease. It lodges in the liver and nibbles its cells over the years. During this phase of 10–20 years, the host has hardly any symptoms and hence does not seek medical attention. When considerable liver damage has resulted in liver cirrhosis (20 per cent develop it), symptoms begin to appear: lethargy, fatigue, swelling of the feet, abdominal distention, or vomiting of blood, drawing attention to this underlying cause. It also increases the risk of developing liver cancer.

There are two common scenarios: One is of a person in his forties who, while undergoing blood tests for a visa application or executive checkup, finds his liver tests (SGPT) to be abnormal, and further tests reveal the cause to be hepatitis C, or tests positive during screening for blood donation. Almost invariably, when asked, they recall having had a blood transfusion, surgery, or injections with non-disposable needles. These people are the lucky ones, as their liver disease is usually not advanced and they stand a good chance of being cured with anti-viral treatment. The other scenario is of a person who presents with symptoms of liver cirrhosis, having had a blood transfusion from a commercial blood bank 20 or more years ago. They do not tolerate treatment well, their disease progresses relentlessly, and they find themselves in need of a liver transplant.

In 20–30 per cent of the cases, hepatitis C is the cause of liver cirrhosis, with alcohol and hepatitis B being the next common causes. Any person who has had a blood transfusion or surgery should get himself tested for this infection, as should anyone whose liver function test shows derangement. Treatment is now easy with the recent launch of the new oral drug called Sofosbuvir, which has to be taken with ribavirin or pegylated interferon injections for three to six months.

There is, unfortunately, no vaccine yet for preventing hepatitis C, unlike hepatitis B. Hence, prevention and early detection assume greater importance. If you have ever received a blood transfusion or undergone surgery, make sure you have got yourself tested for hepatitis C.

Tales of Hepatitis B

Hepatitis B, a viral infection of the liver, has a mixed bag of stories—some of them are good while others are tragic. Here are some lessons from a single family.

Happy Tale 1: If diagnosed on time, you can keep your liver healthy, and protect it from damage.

Anoop (name changed), a 36-year-old software engineer working with a multinational company who was diagnosed with this infection six years ago during a blood screening drive, visited me recently. His blood reports were perfect: the liver functions were absolutely normal, and his fibroscan showed that his liver was as soft and supple as any healthy person's. He was on a daily oral tablet costing a mere Rs. 800 per month, all these years, but there was no trace of any live virus in his blood. When he asked me how long is he expected to live, I said, "As long as elderly people do in India."

Happy Tale 2: You can prevent getting infected with a very effective and affordable vaccine.

His wife and child had tested negative for hepatitis B on blood screening tests and Anoop, on the recommendation of a doctor, had got them to take three shots of the hepatitis B vaccine. Their recent blood tests had shown high titers of protective antibodies. His face lit up when I told him that they were well protected for the rest of their lives from at least one potentially serious disease, i.e., hepatitis B. And could he plan to have another child with the assurance that the infection will not spread to the newborn? He had the green signal.

The earlier concern about high cost is now history. What used to cost Rs. 500 for each shot now costs Rs. 50 or less. It means you can get a lifetime of protection with three doses for as little as Rs. 150.

Tragic tale: Although Anoop was happy with his reports and those of his wife and child, he still finds it impossible to erase the memories of his father's illness and death. They had taken him to a hospital for swelling of the feet, pain, and distention of the abdomen, where his blood tests and ultrasound had shown a shrunken cirrhotic liver with a large cancer in it. The cause, the doctor explained, was the hepatitis B infection that had been going on for years but had not been detected in time.

His end had been agonising. He had become bedridden, groaning with pain most of the time. He had required repeated admissions to the hospital for tapping out fluid from the abdomen and the infusion of expensive medicines. Toward the end, he would lapse intermittently into a coma. Finally, he vomited a large amount of blood, a spectacle that haunts the family to this day.

World Hepatitis Day is celebrated on the 28th of July. It is an occasion when hospitals and NGOs set up camps and offer free testing and vaccination for hepatitis B. Get yourself and your loved ones tested and vaccinated this year.

05

Madhu and Her New Liver

Not everything has a happy ending, and not everything has an ending. But this time, they lived happily ever after!

Madhu (name changed) is in the 19th year of her new life. She had almost reached her end because of her failing liver when, on 14th February 2004, a new liver arrived in Lucknow almost by miracle.

To go back a bit, she had been a healthy homemaker and mother until 1994 when she had an episode of jaundice. Unlike the common ones that come and then go on their own, her liver problem lingered. One doctor after another, one herbal tonic replaced by another, she finally reached an advanced medical centre after four years. Tests revealed that her chronic liver ailment was not due to the common infective viruses B or C but due to a rare condition called autoimmune hepatitis, a condition in which the body's defending cells and immune system start attacking its own organs, in her case, her liver.

Autoimmune hepatitis is somewhat rare; it accounts for two to five per cent of all prolonged cases of hepatitis or liver cirrhosis. Women are affected five times more commonly. It is diagnosed by a set of special blood and liver tests. If detected on time, the disease can be controlled with immune-suppressive medicines like corticosteroids.

Madhu had reached us somewhat late when a major portion of her liver had been permanently damaged. She was treated with immunosuppressive medications to preserve the viable portion of her liver. She had her ups and downs but remained largely healthy for almost eight years. By 2002, her liver had become weak; she had water in her abdomen, swelling in her feet, and side effects of the medicines as well. It became obvious that only a liver transplant could get her back to life and health at that stage.

Her husband, a bank employee, tried all he could; he consulted various liver transplant centres in India, offered to donate a part of his own liver, and took large loans to provide for the increasing costs of her treatment. Unfortunately, he was considered medically unfit to be a liver donor as he had severe fatty liver. With that, almost all hope had disappeared for Madhu.

On 13th March 2004, a man on a ventilator in one of the hospitals in Delhi following an accident was pronounced brain dead. Under such trying circumstances, his relatives gallantly agreed to donate his liver, wherein the liver is extracted from his body to be put into a needy person with a failing liver. Dr. Peush Sahni from AIIMS extracted the liver and flew into Lucknow on the 14th morning. Madhu was taken into the operation theatre of the Sanjay Gandhi Postgraduate Institute of Medical Institute, where Dr. Rajan Saxena and Dr. Peush Sahni transplanted the new liver into Madhu. That indeed was destiny! The relatives of the donor were magnanimous enough not to seek publicity for saving someone else's life and requested anonymity.

Madhu continues to be well 19 years on. Her daughter got married three years ago.

As a token of gratitude, Madhu and her husband have been providing free counselling to patients suffering from liver failure and their relatives facing similar plights for nearly two decades. And their eyes still well up as they recall that miraculous moment when they found a donor.

01

IV. DIABETES

Fighting Diabetes

*With the courage to begin and the discipline to endure,
victory is only a matter of time.*

It could not have been just chance that my cab driver, Mr. Yadav, a large, burly man hailing from my state of Uttar Pradesh, driving me from a hotel in south Mumbai to the airport in the wee hours of the morning got chatty and told me about his recent brush with doctors and disease. When a toe infection he had suffered a few months ago refused to settle with home remedies, he reluctantly visited a doctor, and a blood test showed his fasting blood sugar to be around 300.

The word DIABETES had shaken him. He was the sole breadwinner not just for his wife and two small children who stayed with him in this city but for a large, expanded family in his village home. He had heard that heart and kidney problems often followed diabetes.

It was around this time of our conversation that I noticed we were cruising down the marine drive where a large, well, actually very large, number of people were thronging the path bordering the sea and spilling onto the beaches.

The city of Paris, I had heard, never sleeps. But this was Mumbai at 6 a.m. As though sensing my question, Mr. Yadav said, "These paths at these times used to be deserted ten years ago. Now they are all here for fear of diabetes!"

I saw people of all ages and both sexes indulging in a variety of workouts: jogging, walking, stretching their bodies, and allowing themselves to be dragged by their pet dogs to a healthy start to another day. Their faces were, as is usual with *Mumbaikars*, intense in their singular pursuits rather than the cheerful, vibrant ones in Lucknow. But kudos to them; they were at it from dawn, trying to shed their excess baggage of fat, pacing up their hearts, improving their stamina, and trying to ward off the dreaded diabetes.

Mr. Yadav went on to say, "Sir, I lost ten kg over three months too and brought my weight down from 110 to 100 kg, by cutting down on sweets and walking five km every day. My sugar came down, and the wound healed."

To my unasked question, "What happened thereafter?", he replied, "I stopped my exercise and gained back three kg."

Does he regret it? He seemed somewhat torn between the conventional advice of *aaram (rest)* from elders in his village and the *push yourself, run, and shed weight* that *Mumbaikars* practice and preach.

As we neared the airport, he bowled me a final spinner and asked, "What do you do, Sir?"

I am lazy by nature, and getting up early for exercise, or, for that matter, to catch morning flights has always been my worst punishment.

As we parted at the airport, we both felt united by our roots and traits and secretly resolved to shelve our traditional laziness and restart a daily dose of workouts in our own lives and cities to keep the common enemy of diabetes at bay.

02

Diabetes and the Liver

To study the phenomenon of disease without books is to sail an uncharted sea, while to study books without patients is not to go to sea at all. – Sir William Osler

One could wonder why, in diabetes, a condition in which the blood sugar level goes up, we need to worry about the liver. Or, for that matter, even take the blood sugar reports seriously.

Doctors have begun to realise that the elevated blood sugar value is only the tip of the iceberg. Patients with type 2 diabetes, the common form of the disease that occurs in adulthood, often go on to develop problems with several other organs of the body, such as the kidneys, brain, blood vessels, heart, feet, and liver.

At the root of the problem in type 2 diabetes is the question, "Why do the blood sugar levels go up?" The intuitive answer would be a shortage of the hormone called insulin, which is produced by the pancreas and does the job of driving blood sugar levels down. Contrary to expectations, the blood sugar levels in this condition are usually increased.

The answer is, therefore, complex, but it starts with the recognition of the underlying condition called Insulin Resistance (IR). One finds that as time goes on, some people need higher and higher amounts of insulin in the blood to push the blood glucose into cells and keep the sugar in check.

This is in contrast to type 1 diabetes, which is caused by a shortfall in insulin production. But the common type 2 diabetes is characterised, at least in its early stages, by not just high blood sugar levels but also high insulin levels.

IR brings with it several changes in the body, such as the thickening of the basement membrane, the floor on which cells of all organs of the body are lined up, and pushes up fatty acids in blood circulation, which then get deposited in the liver and blood vessels.

Diabetes, therefore, affects several organs of the body and does not usually come alone. It can be associated with obesity, increased blood lipids (cholesterol or triglycerides), and high blood pressure, all of which can be caused by IR as the underlying mechanism.

Diabetes affecting the kidneys, eyes, feet, and heart is now common knowledge. Its effects on the liver often go unnoticed.

Fatty liver is very commonly seen in patients with type 2 diabetes and can be picked up by a simple ultrasound examination in up to 70 per cent of them. This condition results from the excess accumulation of fat in liver cells. The liver is usually enlarged and is pale and greasy to see.

Fatty liver usually has no clear symptoms in the early stages. It is diagnosed during investigations for abnormal readings on liver function tests (AST, ALT, or GGT levels in blood) or during an ultrasound examination.

A more reliable new test that is quick, accurate, and painless is the latest version of liver fibroscan with CAP. This machine uses low-frequency ultrasound waves and, through a new technology, is able to measure the amount of fat in the liver. It scores over ultrasound as the latter cannot quite give a definite idea, and whether it is mild or severe often depends upon the impression of the sonographer.

There are other tests to estimate liver fat, too. The time-tested method has been liver biopsy; this procedure is painful and requires hospitalisation for a day. Other methods include a special version of MRI that uses spectroscopy to measure fat. The fibroscan has, however, emerged as the simplest and easiest one.

Although fatty liver disease does not produce many symptoms in the early stages, and sometimes even the blood tests for liver function are normal, it is not an innocuous condition. Research shows that patients with extra fat in their livers die earlier; that is, their lives are shorter than their fat-free counterparts.

What damage does liver fat do? Some of them go on to develop a state of weakness in the liver called liver cirrhosis. In this condition, liver cells die insidiously and are replaced by scar tissue. The organ gradually starts functioning poorly, sometimes causing swelling of the feet or retention of water in the abdomen. The veins in the food pipe can get engorged and rupture, causing blood vomiting.

When the liver gets very weak due to liver cirrhosis, transplantation of the diseased organ is sometimes required. This condition is getting so common that it makes up around a third of all causes of liver transplantation.

Why the disease progresses rapidly in some and slowly in others is not always evident. Understandably, those who also have other contributory factors such as obesity, excess alcohol consumption, hypertension, or elevated blood cholesterol levels are more likely to progress rapidly. But doctors still do not know for sure why some seem to progress more rapidly while others seem to remain stable for years.

The advent of liver fibroscan has made a significant change in the way patients with fatty livers are evaluated nowadays. The estimation of fat content is the starting point. Those with very high values need to work hard to get their livers in shape.

The test also measures the stiffness of the liver at the same time and tells whether scarring of the organ has begun. If indeed it has, one needs to get serious and work hard to make sure that the disease does not progress to the stage of liver failure, requiring a liver transplant.

Another recent finding that research has shown is that patients with diabetes and fatty livers are at increased risk of developing liver cancer. They often come silently or are incidentally picked up on imaging tests, but progress aggressively over a few months. Scientists are debating whether all type 2 diabetics with excess fat in their liver should be monitored periodically with CT scans or MRI scans to watch for early liver cancer.

Diabetics also develop stones in their gallbladders more frequently. It is best to have them removed by laparoscopic surgery before they cause pain or complications.

Conclusion:

Diabetics are very prone to developing fatty liver. This condition, earlier thought to be innocuous, has now been seen to progress to liver cirrhosis or liver cancer in a significant proportion of patients. Good control of diabetes with diet, exercise, and medications and the maintenance of proper body weight reduce the risk. Screening programs with newer tests help detect and treat liver problems better if done periodically.

03

Gut Woes in Diabetics

They muddy the water and make it seem deep.
– Friedrich Nietzsche

Of the many adverse effects that diabetes has on the body, a troublesome one is the increased frequency of visits to the washroom, to pass stools, in some. Diabetics are almost twice more likely to suffer from loose, frequent stools, compared to their non-diabetic counterparts.

A recent study conducted on over 1,500 diabetics found that 15 to 30 per cent of diabetics reported diarrhoea (more than three stools per day or loose stools). It was more common in those whose sugars were poorly controlled and in those who have had diabetes for a long.

The reasons are many and vary from simple triggers to more complex issues.

- Some of the medicines and food additives that diabetics take can cause diarrhoea. These include some artificial sweeteners, such as sucralose, and medicines, such as metformin and acarabose.
- Celiac disease, an immune sensitivity to a component of wheat called gluten, is more common in diabetics, especially younger ones. It usually manifests as diarrhoea, anaemia, and growth failure in childhood but could manifest in its 'adult' avatar in adult diabetics too. A simple blood test helps settle the issue.

- Another important cause is a condition called small intestinal bacterial overgrowth, nicknamed SIBO. In this condition, the small intestine, which is normally sparsely colonised by bacteria, is somewhat overloaded with a copious number of bugs that break down food, interfering with digestion and absorption.
- Diabetic autonomic neuropathy is another important and specific cause of intestinal dysfunction that occurs in long-standing diabetics with poor control of sugars. In this condition, the nerves get weak and damaged, leading to poor regulation of bowel movements. It usually does not come alone and is associated with other forms of autonomic malfunction, such as postural hypotension (giddiness on standing up from a lying position), poor bladder control, unsteadiness of gait, and so on.
- It is, however, important to keep in mind that all other causes of diarrhoea that occur in a non-diabetic could occur in a diabetic as well. Common infections in India include amoeba, giardia, shigella, salmonella, and cryptospora. They need to be treated when found or suspected.
- The two varieties of inflammatory bowel disease—ulcerative colitis and Crohn's disease—can occur in people with diabetes. The diagnosis requires an examination of the stool, blood, and intestines. It is also prudent to remember that colon cancer, which becomes more common with age, could also occur in a diabetic.
- Another problem that becomes more frequent with ageing is poorly coordinated rectal contractions to expel stools fully, or defecation disorders, as they are called. Diagnosis and treatment with biofeedback can be very helpful.
- Not to be overlooked is the common problem of IBS, a condition in which the bowels move with greater enthusiasm

and vigour than one would have liked. It should be diagnosed with caution only after the list above has been checked and excluded.

Diarrhoea in diabetics could indeed be a clinical challenge for diagnosis and management, but awareness could be the key.

04

Reversing Diabetes with Fasting

One does not discover new lands without consenting to lose sight of the shore for a very long time. – Andre Gide

There is some cheer from the research world for diabetics. A recent experiment has shown that diabetes, a disease that is considered irreversible and progressive through one's lifetime, can be reversed. The pancreas, especially its beta cells that produce insulin, may be coaxed to regenerate, thus reversing diabetes.

Dr. Valter Longo and colleagues from the University of South California, USA, who published their findings in the prestigious journal Cell, showed that the pancreas of diabetic mice could be made to regenerate with a special type of fasting diet.

What seems to be doing the trick is that fasting gives the pancreas some respite from a continuous barrage of calories demanding more and more production of insulin from a fatigued gland, giving it time to recuperate instead.

In their experiment, diabetic mice were put on a 'fasting-mimicking diet' for a few months. The diet was low in calories, carbohydrates, and proteins but high in unsaturated fats. The periods of starvation were alternated with 25 eat-what-you-want days. To their surprise, the mice showed marked improvement in diabetes as well as beta cell function.

Dr. Valter Longo said, "Our conclusion is that by pushing the mice into an extreme state and then bringing them back—by starving them and then feeding them again—the cells in the pancreas are triggered to use some kind of developmental reprogramming that rebuilds the part of the organ that is no longer functioning."

The emerging pandemic of diabetes seems to be related to the ingestion of excess calories by genetically predisposed individuals. It leads initially to IR, where the hormone finds it hard to drive and metabolise glucose in cells, in turn stimulating its increased production in the pancreas. Over time, the gland gets exhausted, and insulin production drops off.

Fasting, or, for that matter, starving, seems to help re-boot the pancreas. Several studies have shown that people who fast periodically have lower chances of developing diabetes. During both world wars, the mortality rate from diabetes dropped precipitously. In the interwar period, as people went back to their accustomed eating habits, they went back up.

The reason why this news has perhaps not made as big headlines as one would have expected is probably because the therapeutic formula for regenerating the pancreas is neither a drug marketed by a pharmaceutical house nor a patented fad diet promoted online.

After the discovery of insulin in the early 1920s, all the focus turned to it as the cure for diabetes. While it was a major advance for type 1, it was not quite the panacea for type 2 diabetes. However, most of the interest in fasting disappeared as doctors focused on what would be their mantra for the next century—drugs, drugs, and more drugs.

With Navratri, Ramzan, or, for that matter, any occasion you wish to choose, you could make periodic fasting a promising remedy for the new-age malady.

V. MISCELLANY

Life must be understood backwards, but it must be lived forwards.
– Soren Kierkegaard

Heads will Ache

Maturity is realising how many things do not require your opinion.

Headaches are so common that not to have ever suffered from it raises doubts whether the head is indeed there. While most are innocuous and transient and pass away with time or with a painkiller, some could be indicators of worrisome underlying problems.

The head often aches when other parts of the body are under strain. It accompanies seasonal fevers and fasts and often appears after a gruelling day under the hot sun. It is not uncommon after a sleepless night of exam preparation, international travel, or watching the last of the day's FIFA World Cup matches. The heads of young women often ache before or during periods. It can also be brought about by mental stress such as a rebuke by the boss, a spat at work, or a feud at home.

Migraine is a common but specific form of headache that occurs due to spasms of arteries in the head. In its typical pattern, these attacks start with a mild ache starting in one-half of the head, often associated with visual auras such as light flashes or sparkling lights. Over hours it progresses to intense throbbing pain in the head, often associated with nausea, vomiting, and restlessness. Painkillers don't work at this stage. Falling asleep often terminates the attack but some patients have it going for a day or two.

Migraine sufferers often learn to recognise what triggers their attacks (menstrual periods, fasts, bright sunlight, lack of sleep, red wine or cheese, physical or emotional stress, etc.) as well as the early phase of an episode, as a painkiller pill popped in at this time helps abort a full-blown throbbing attack. Avoiding the triggers helps reduce the episodes too. If they are disablingly frequent and intense, mild medicines such as propranolol or Sibelium are very helpful. Yoga and positive lifestyle changes, if pursued regularly, often provide much relief.

Unlike most stress-related headaches that come on by the end of the day, early morning headaches have a different connotation. When they occur in hypertensive patients they suggest that the BP is poorly controlled. In a diabetic, they indicate that the blood sugar levels are dropping too low at night (nocturnal hypoglycaemia). Although rare, patients with increased pressure within their heads from causes such as tumours also complain of morning headaches, often accompanied by vomiting.

The age also matters. Headache in a school child is often due to eyesight disorders such as short-sightedness, stuffy choked ears, or a blocked nose. Pain from sinusitis is usually located toward the front and gets worse with head movements.

In the middle or older ages, cervical spondylosis is a common cause, especially if the ache tends to radiate down to the neck and back and worsens with movements of the neck.

Analysing, diagnosing, and treating headaches can be a challenge to doctors as well. A detailed clinical evaluation often holds the key that an expensive MRI scan cannot provide. And a gentle massage of the aching head by the spouse often achieves what the strongest painkillers fail at!

02

Obesity, Are Genes Partly Responsible?

Regardless of your metabolism, if you stop consuming so many calories, you will lose weight. – Rob McElhenney.

If you are battling excess body weight and feeling frustrated with the weighing machine needle stubbornly refusing to move left despite all the starvation and workouts, here are some new facts to console you.

A global survey has reported that the number of obese people across the globe is a whopping two billion, outstripping starvation for the first time in numerical terms.

A quick catching up for those joining in and still not familiar with BMI, it is a measure of how your weight relates to your height and is calculated by dividing your weight (in kg) by your height (in metres squared). If you are not good with math, just put your weight and height on any of the calculators available on the net, and you will have your BMI.

A healthy BMI value should be between 20 and 25 (preferably below 23.5 for Indians). Those with values between 25 to 30 are overweight. If the BMI crosses 30 the term obesity is used. A value between 35 to 40 puts the person in a category called severe obesity, while above 40 is called morbid obesity, indicating a major risk of early death.

There is still debate whether obesity should be called a disease as history tells us that people who had extra fat reserves survived famines better in earlier times. Hence, if it was an advantage up until 20 years ago, it could not have become a disease so soon.

The difference between earlier and present times, however, is that prolonged periods of starvation do not occur to many anymore; hence the body does not get a chance to shed the excess energy that it accumulated gradually over days, months, and years.

Scientists have suspected the role of certain genes, fancily termed 'thrifty genes' that could be causing energy pile up in some individuals. Why should only a few of several people eating the same quality and quantity of food start bulging while others remain slim? They could well be harbouring genes that make them conserve energy in the body in the form of fat.

One candidate gene of the class of fat mass and obesity associated gene (FTO gene) that has been recently identified in humans is called PNPLA3. A variant of it has been linked to not just extra fat accumulation in the body, but to its deposition in the liver and risk to life due to liver and heart diseases.

Our genetic predisposition is sometimes evident when you simply look at a family photograph or obtain a family history. Children of obese or overweight parent(s) often tend to become like their parents; if both are obese, the propensity is higher, with family attitudes towards eating and fitness patterns chipping in.

While our genetic make up is what we inherit, and is not possible to change, knowing helps us strategize our special needs, strategies, and goals.

03

Skeletal Muscle: Latest Member to Join the Endocrine Club

Progress is impossible without change, and those who cannot change their minds cannot change anything.
– George Bernard Shaw

Hormones, or chemical proteins that circulate in the blood and regulate body function, have long been known to be produced by just a handful of endocrine glands such as the pituitary, thyroid, parathyroid, adrenals, pancreas, and gonads. The three latest ones to join this exclusive club are intestines, bones, and skeletal muscles.

It may sound funny but medical scientists are beginning to discover how some of these large tissues also produce hormones and regulate metabolism.

Skeletal muscles, for instance, produce a wide variety of hormones, largely referred to as myokines. Their subtle actions range from maintaining blood sugar levels (apart from insulin), keeping us in a good mood (stretching skeletal muscles has stress-busting effects on the brain), improving fat metabolism (converts white fat to brown fat and reducing its quantity), improving liver functions, regulating bowel movements, and removing cholesterol plaques from blood vessels.

What goes on between myokines and other organ systems is referred to in scientific circles, as CROSS TALK. The myokines released from muscle fibres during exercise or stretching, interact with other systems and hormones. Some of the important functions recently ascribed to myokines are improved cognition (alertness, learning), anti-depressive, reduced stress hormone levels, and cardio-protection.

To make it simple, research is showing that those who have been actively exercising are less prone to fatty liver disease and developing diabetes. Their tendency to develop Alzheimer's disease is less and demonstrate less risk of developing cancers.

The discovery came in the year 2000 when it was discovered that exercise caused the release of a hormone-like substance called IL-6 (interleukin 6) from muscles into the circulation. It turns out that this IL-6 has anti-inflammatory and health-promoting properties that it exerts on several organs, from the brain to the liver.

The only way to get your share of IL-6 release into the circulation, unfortunately, is by stretching, doing some exercise, and squeezing your muscles to release it. This set of observations now explains why healthy living requires a daily dose of myokines or IL-6, and no pill can help provide that as of now.

04

Thyroid Disorders

Intellect takes you to the door, but it does not take you into the house. – Shams Tabirzi

One of the three common causes of poor performance of students in schools and colleges has been ascribed to insufficient functioning of a small gland situated in the front of our neck, called the thyroid. While weighing only around 50 grams, the thyroid gland produces the hormone thyroxin which regulates how our body functions, or its metabolism.

As the role of the hormone is to pace up the body and mind and keep us active and alert, its low production leads to just the opposite: dullness, lethargy, sluggishness, drowsiness, lack of concentration, and obesity.

Indeed it is this dullness and lethargy that makes poor learners and performers of students. The role of the thyroid is often overlooked and the blame is placed on other factors such as the role of parents, distractions by television, or even the quality of teachers.

There are several ways and phases in which hypothyroidism, or inadequate function of the gland, may present itself. It presents as cretinism in infants and small children. These kids are stunted in growth, have coarse skin, are retarded mentally, and show growth failure. A deficiency of iodine is often the underlying cause.

When it manifests in adults, especially women, the signs are often subtle, with increasing weight, fatigue, heavy infrequent periods, cold intolerance, high blood pressure, increased levels of cholesterol, hoarseness of voice, coarse skin, loss of eyebrows, or even depression, in isolation or combination. Some may also have a goitre or prominent swelling of the gland in the neck, due to long-term deficiency of iodine.

Thyroid problems are indeed common in adults with 10-30 per cent showing evidence of dysfunction when tested.

Detecting Hypothyroidism is easy. A simple blood test that estimates TSH (thyroid stimulating hormone) tells you where you stand. In early hypothyroidism, TSH values (normal 1-5) are increased above normal limits, demonstrating that more pressure is required by TSH to flog a tired thyroid gland to produce thyroxin. With the further progressive weakness of the gland, thyroxin levels start falling despite TSH levels climbing further.

Once detected, treatment is quite easy and requires the hormone to be taken every day as replenishment. The daily dose, best taken in the early morning on an empty stomach, needs to be titrated by the doctor. Improvement is usually obvious in weeks, with friends often noticing a change in appearance and personality.

A rarer form of thyroid disorder is one in which the gland produces an excess of the hormone, called hyperthyroidism. It presents as prominent bulging eyes, rapid pulse rate, weight loss, and excessive sweating. Treatment here aims at slowing down the overactive thyroid gland.

Thyroid disorders are often so indefinable and subtle in their signs and yet have such far-reaching effects on the functions of our body, mind, and personality that experts recommend testing them as a part of general checkups. And with treatment being so simple and rewarding, the stakes of missing it are indeed high.

Section F

Cancer Today

Not everything that is faced can be changed,
but nothing can be changed until it is faced.
– James Baldwin

01

The Kylie Factor

Once I overcame breast cancer, I wasn't afraid of anything anymore. – Melissa Etheridge

Kylie Minogue, the sultry Australian pop singer and actress, was detected to have breast cancer at the age of 37. The diagnosis forced this international celebrity to put an end to her Showgirl Tour and career. She underwent breast surgery in Melbourne in May 2005, followed by chemotherapy in France. What makes her so special is the way she underwent treatment for her disease under an intense public gaze and the openness with which she shared her experience with her fans and the public. She is back on track in her career, where she is flying even higher than before.

Voted 'Woman of the Year' in 2006 because of her inspirational fight against the disease, Kylie helped create a wave of awareness among fans and the public about breast cancer. It led to a spike in screening tests in women. Described as the 'Kylie Factor', 40 per cent more women underwent mammography and other tests as part of a cancer detection checkup.

Breast cancer is the most common cancer in women in developed countries, afflicting one in every eight. It is the second most common cancer (cancer of the cervix being the most common) in India and is estimated to occur in one in every 22 women. Around 80,000 women are diagnosed with this condition in India every year. It usually occurs in the fourth to seventh decade but may occur in younger age, as was the case with Kylie Minogue. Women with a family history of breast or uterine cancer, those who have not borne babies, and Parsis are at high risk. Mutation of the genes (BRCA1 and BRCA2) accounts for the development of this cancer in a significant proportion of cases.

Breast cancer is curable if diagnosed at an early stage when it is usually painless. This underscores the need for greater awareness of women. It can be picked up by regular routine self-examination of the breast and a mammography test in those above 45. Treatment consists of the removal of the small lump by surgery, followed by some medications. The breast does not always have to be removed fully or can be reconstructed for cosmetic reasons.

Treatment is more difficult if the disease is diagnosed at an advanced stage, especially when it has spread to other parts of the body. Surgery, even extensive, may not succeed in removing the entire tumour and chemotherapy may not be able to kill all the cancer cells. The outcome in this setting remains somewhat grim.

Kylie had likened her cancer battle to 'experiencing a nuclear bomb', but has fought and won it with grit and determination. As a pop legend, she has sold more than 60 million records. She has, however, become immortal in creating awareness about breast cancer in women.

02

Removing Breasts Before Cancer Strikes

An ounce of cancer prevention is worth a ton of cancer cure.
– Robert A Wascher

Angelina Jolie's decision to put both her normal healthy breasts under the knife as a precaution against the possibility of developing cancer has evoked a flutter in both medical and women's worlds.

This bold step taken by the Hollywood actress and international celebrity has left many wondering how far is far enough, not just to treat diseases, but to undergo aggressive interventions to reduce the risks of their occurring. The coin obviously has two sides.

No doubt, breast cancer is the most common cancer in women in developed countries, afflicting one in every eight, and despite advancements in diagnosis and treatment, still remains a major killer. Women with a family history of breast or uterine cancer are at particularly high risk by often inheriting faulty genes such as BRCA1 and BRCA2 that predispose them.

Angelina had these: her mother had breast cancer, and her own genetic testing had shown that she harboured the dangerous gene, putting her at 87 per cent risk of developing the disease in her lifetime. And as it is not possible to speculate which one of the two breasts it might occur in, precautionary removal, if needed, had to be of both.

In the surgery she underwent, tissue was scooped out through a small incision from each of her breasts, which were then filled with implants to make them look cosmetically 'normal'.

Genetic testing, such as that of cancer-causing genes of breast, uterus, or colon is beginning to come of age. Scientists argue that those with a strong family history of these cancers should get themselves tested, and have their risks profiled.

Removal of an organ to ward off cancer is now getting popular. In a rare genetic disorder called familial adenomatous polyposis in which the large intestine is studded with polyps, and that almost invariably turn cancerous by age 20, prophylactic colectomy offers the only hope of long-term survival and is strongly recommended.

On the other side of the coin, genetic testing especially for breast cancer is still an evolving field. The test is not easily available, is exorbitantly priced, and barring a few instances, competes with astrology in predicting bad times through probability. Further, it encroaches far beyond its organ such as the breast, to that of human feelings and fears.

Biomedical scientists need to keep in mind the emotional consequences of testing too. How would a woman who undertakes the test and comes positive, when told she has a very high risk of coming down with cancer, be expected to react? Wouldn't fear blind her to the small 13 per cent chance of not getting cancer?

The line that divides informing patients about their risk and frightening them is often thin and blurred.

However, having seen her mother and grandmother suffer from the deadly disease, and with science putting her at an 87% risk of developing the disease, her choice has been hailed as logical and scientifically sound.

03

Cancer Takes the Final Bow

It always seems impossible until it is done. - Nelson Mandela

The ovation that marked Yuvraj Singh's return to the cricket field has much more to do than just a cricketer's homecoming to the lime-lit pitch. It has come to symbolise human triumph over a disease that has till now been considered invariably fatal.

Yuvi's rendezvous with the rare germ-cell cancer, starting from its delayed diagnosis, his hesitation to confront it and start treatment, the bewildering experience of seeing his bald head in the mirror, and his anguish of having to sit away while his team played on the field have made his cancer a touching human story for the public. And, in our all too familiar Bollywood style of *All's well that ends well*, his return to the cricket field with hair on his head gives us the *deja vu* feeling of the climax when the villain is finally bashed up by the hero.

Our perception of cancer has been undergoing considerable change over the last few decades. Rajesh Khanna's epic movie, Anand, depicted it as a tragic illness that ultimately took its toll. Fighting it was not much of an option, and going down gracefully was all that one could do.

Kylie Minogue's affliction with breast cancer in the last decade rang a similar bell as that of Yuvi's and made women both aware and confident about dealing with a disease that has haunted them. This Australian celebrity pop singer's untimely detection of breast cancer, her long fight with the disease, her candid disclosures of her illness, and her final victory over it heralded by her return to the stage helped convince many that this too was possible.

Five South American leaders have been diagnosed with cancer. And as is the spirit of our modern times, they are all battling it well and continuing to lead their nations. Fidel Castro, the veteran Cuban leader, was the eldest and most senior one to undergo surgery for his disease. Hugo Chavez, the outspoken Venezuelan president has undergone several surgeries for his cancer and has been probably certified cured. Argentina's elegant lady leader Christina Fernandez de Kirchner had thyroid cancer, from which she has recovered. Two of Brazil's leaders, the current president Luiz Inacio Lula de Silva, and the past president Dilma Rousseff are cancer patients. And in neighbouring Paraguay, Fernando Lugo is battling cancer too.

Cancer is no longer a disease that is rare and occurs only in others. It has found its way from remote corners to the backyards and now to our homes. What, however, has changed in recent times is our spirit—from an easily yielding one in Anand to that of an indomitable and resilient one, fuelled by our resolve to return to the field to play again.

04

Cancer Survivor Wins Olympic Gold Medal

Every champion was also once a contender.

If 'cancer' and 'chemotherapy' evoke fear and hopelessness in you, you must read this.

Canada's 27-year-old Max Parrot soared to victory at the Beijing Winter Olympics in the snowboard competition, enthralling many watchers with his flying antics and winning the gold medal.

Five years ago, Max was diagnosed with Hodgkin's Lymphoma, when he noticed a lump in the neck. It is a type of cancer of the body's immune cells that occurs in lymph glands.

The mainstay of therapy for this group of cancers is chemotherapy, where several cycles of drugs are administered into the body to target and kill the cancerous cells.

Not unexpectedly, he described 2018 as a year when he felt to be at zero level, fighting not just his cancer, but the adverse effects of therapy. He describes his experience as, "lying in a hospital with no energy, no muscles, and no cardio."

For an active sportsman, the interruption in his career, mental trauma, and disappointment is not hard to imagine.

Over the past few decades, cancer treatment has moved from the almost 'invariably progressive and fatal' to a good deal of success. According to the American Cancer Society, the chances of long-term survival of patients with Hodgkin's Lymphoma (measured as five-year survival rates) have moved up to 90 per cent. In other words, nine of every ten patients are expected to respond and survive five years. Even more reassuring is that most who do, are often cured for life.

As for Max, the treatment comprising 12 cycles of chemotherapy was exhausting. What kept him going were probably his young age and desire to get back on the snowboard, his favourite sport.

Within a few months after his therapy, he had started training again. And many people, including his Canadian friend and colleague who won the bronze medal, were happy that he managed to prove himself.

Section G

Sleep and Brain Disorders

A new challenge keeps the brain kicking and the heart ticking.
– E A Ponchiqueri

01

Sleep and Dreams

Dreams say what they mean, but they don't say it in daytime language. – Gail Godwin

Dreams are an essential component of good sleep, and if you are not dreaming enough, it could be that your sleep is not of the quality that you deserve.

Do you remember what you dreamed of last night? Even if you can't and are under the impression that your sleep was dreamless, you would have dreamed more than two hours or 25 per cent of the time that you slept.

Dreams are successions of images, ideas, emotions, and sensations occurring involuntarily in the mind during certain stages of sleep. Good or bad, dreams always take us to some interesting places. They can range from normal to surreal and bizarre. Dreams can at times spring a creative thought or give a sense of inspiration. Dream imagery is usually absurd and unrealistic and they are generally outside the control of the dreamer. They can vary from frightening, exciting, magical, and melancholic to adventurous.

Dreaming is as old as human history; it finds mention in ancient Mesopotamian, Chinese, Assyrian, Greek, and Indian texts. Credit for the first serious attempt to study and understand dreams, called Oneirology, goes to the European scientist-philosopher Sigmund Freud, who described it as "the royal road to the unconscious mind when we lose our consciousness during sleep."

Men and women probably dream just as much but women tend to remember dreams better, especially during pregnancy. Several factors influence dreams of which smell is particularly important. People exposed to the smell of rotten eggs while sleeping, report bad dreams when woken up. On the other hand, the smell of roses during sleep produces pleasant dreams.

Sound also affects the quality of dreams. The sound of falling water often results in dreams of swimming or seas, and can often trigger bed wetting, as often happens when it rains at night. A child sleeps well when a soothing lullaby is sung to him.

Bad dreams are not uncommon and often take the form of falling or being chased. They generate a lot of anxiety and may wake you up with panic and sweat. They are common when the body or the mind is in pain, when the external stimuli such as smell and sound are unpleasant, during indigestion, and when the blood sugar drops during sleep as in some diabetics on insulin. It is also associated with the use of certain medications like propranolol or barbiturates. Dreams of choking and strangulation are common when suffering from a blocked nose, or chest infection, or during passive smoking.

Good sleep, of which dream is an essential part, helps our brain to regulate mood, solve problems, reduce stress, and feel refreshed. Dreamless sleep, as happens with certain sleeping drugs or under the effect of alcohol, lacks these benefits.

Your dreams could tell you much about the state of your health. If you are getting pleasant dreams, you are probably physically well, getting adequate sleep, and are in a stable state of mind. If you are getting recurrent bad dreams, there is something that is desperately trying to draw your attention. Listen to it!

02

Sleep is Emerging as a New Risk Factor for Heart Disease

A ruffled mind makes a restless pillow. – Charlotte Bronte

Adequate sleep, both in terms of duration and quality, is proving to be essential for heart health. The relationship may be a complicated one though. Excess sleep of more than nine hours is harmful, and may understandably make the body sluggish and vulnerable.

However, those sleeping less than seven hours a day on average have been found to have a higher possibility of heart disease.

The healthy sleep duration, therefore, seems to be between seven and eight hours. And early risers fare somewhat better than late ones.

The quality of sleep also seems to clearly matter: those with sleep apnoea (orthostatic sleep apnoea), snoring problems, and sleeping disorders such as difficulty in falling asleep or waking up frequently at night, suffer more frequently from heart ailments.

Which then are the 'types' of heart ailments associated with unhealthy sleep? Heart attack rates are clearly up, as are rates of heart failure and coronary artery disease.

Experts attribute the increased cardiac risk to higher blood pressure levels and increased levels of certain hormones circulating during the night, particularly in people with sleeping problems.

Cardiac disease is the largest killer in urban India today, and doctors as well as patients are familiar with the seven conventional risk factors: tobacco, high BP, high cholesterol, diabetes, strong family history, lack of exercise, and obesity. Sleep is on the threshold of joining in as the eighth risk factor for cardiac diseases.

Interestingly, some of the risk factors are intricately interrelated, and may not be so difficult to handle. Adequate physical exercise, for example, could additionally solve the problem of being overweight as well as lack of sleep, apart from being protective of the heart.

What then prevents you from catching seven hours of good sleep every night? Late-night parties, television, or late hours at work? Sleep therapists strongly advise an early light dinner, and switching off all electronic devices (TV and cellphones) at least an hour before sleeping time. It could be worth following their advice to protect your heart.

03

Natural Ways to Get Sleep

The best bridge between despair and hope is a good night's sleep.
– E Joseph Cossman

It is funny that while sleep is a natural state of relaxation in which we spend one-third of our day or a third of our total life, many of us seem to struggle to get it.

Sleep, in contrast to wakefulness, is a condition when our conscious mind switches off and drifts to the stage of the unconscious mind that often reveals itself in the form of dreams. Healthy sleep in adequate amounts is essential for our brains, minds, and bodies.

Popping a sleeping pill has become an easy way out. At the last count, there are over a hundred types of sleeping pills available for treating insomnia, the medical term for lack of sleep, with three in every 20 Indians consuming them. Most medications provide an abnormal drugged form of sleep which creates dependence on them or has adverse effects.

Getting enough natural sleep at the appropriate time, therefore, continues to be a challenge.

The most common form of sleep disorder especially in young people is difficulty in falling asleep. It is sometimes due to excess consumption of caffeine, a cerebral stimulant, especially in the evenings. Saying no to coffee, tea, and chocolates, especially after dusk helps.

Another form of cerebral stimulation that interferes with sleep is watching thriller movies or heated arguments on television before bedtime. Therefore, though I like watching 'What the Nation Wants to Know', I have started tuning in to 'Bhabiji ghar par hai' to get into the right mood to fall asleep. Working on computers at night can drive sleep away too.

A dark silent cool room without mosquitoes and a comfortable bed often suffice. Additional sleep inducers could be soft instrumental music, *bhajans* or lullabies, or soothing aromas. Reading a book can be an effective strategy for some.

What do you do if these simple measures are not enough?

The strategy that works best for me is physical exercise. On days that I am able to get a 30-minute session of tennis, shuttle, or brisk walk, I find myself dosing off by ten even when mud-fest on TV is reaching deafening levels.

Two other simple tricks also work well.

One is to relax all muscles of the body, working up stepwise from the toes to the forehead, making sure that the body is loose and limp. Direct the mind to the slowing and relaxing rhythm of breathing. Then focus the mind on a soothing scene. What works for me is to visualise sheep grazing on the hilly Himalayan meadow while I try to count them. Another sleep-inducing mental exercise is to subtract seven from 100 and count backwards.

Falling asleep requires wiping off excitement, fears, and anger, and shutting off the conscious mind to let the body go limp and loose into that dream-like state. The more one practices, the easier it gets. And saying a silent prayer often improves the quality of the mist that wafts in.

04

Brain Fog

When life is foggy, the path is unclear, and the mind is dull, remember your breath. It has the power to give you the peace. It has the power to resolve the unsolved equations of life.
– Amit Ray

Fogginess of the brain is a frequently reported symptom these days and can be best described as:

- Cloudy thinking
- Inability to concentrate the way that one could
- Lapses in memory
- Losing train of thought such as forgetting in mid-sentence what you were planning to say, or asking the other person, *What was I saying,* frequently
- Getting distracted easily, with the feeling that the mind is refusing to focus
- Poor motivation

We all experience these symptoms once in a while, but if they become disturbing enough to be noticed and affect the quality of life and work, you could be suffering from Brain Fog.

Reporting of Brain Fog has gone up significantly since the COVID pandemic. It is included as one of the features of long-COVID or post-COVID syndrome.

It is now well-recognised that the COVID-19 virus may cause inflammation or swelling of several organs and tissues. The main brunt has been on the lungs but the involvement of other organs has thrown up their own typical signs in their own ways such as heart (heart attacks), liver (increased liver enzymes), intestines (abdominal pain or diarrhoea), and brain (loss of smell).

It is, therefore, possible that another milder but less dramatic form of brain inflammation could produce the symptoms of Brain Fog, that could last long.

Brain Fog may, however, occur in people who have not had COVID, too.

If persistent, one could run through the checklist.

- Check your blood sugar, blood pressure, haemoglobin, vitamin B12, and vitamin D levels
- Look out for hormonal changes, especially irregularity of periods or thyroid dysfunction
- Are you overworked, stressed out, or sleep-deprived?
- Are you on medications for sleep or depression? Are you consuming alcohol?

For a start, try:

- Seven to nine hours of sleep daily for a few days
- Caffeine could help: Try a cup of coffee or tea to stimulate your brain
- Exercise: A daily dose of 30 minutes of cardio could improve blood circulation to the brain

If the symptoms persist, other possible underlying conditions could be:

- Air pollution (try a vacation to the hills or get an air purifier and use it, especially at night)

- Depression, especially if you experience recurrent negative thoughts, irritability, and low moods
- Early onset of dementia could be a worry, but fortunately, most people improve with the above measures and gain back their brain's vitality.

05

Dementia

The disease may hide the person underneath, but there is still a person in there who needs your love and attention.
– Jamie Calandriello

If you have taken your elderly relative to the doctor, the conversation can go sometimes like this:

"Can you tell me which year are we in? Season? Day? Month? Thank you.

Could you tell me where we are? Town? Country? Good.

Now name the three things I am pointing at (pencil, paperweight, paper). Thanks.

Could you count backwards from 100 by sevens? Yes, Please try. 93, good, then…

Earlier I showed you three things. Can you remember them?"

And although heartbreaking, you would realise that the doctor is trying to assess whether your relative's mind has started to slow or even slip.

As we are living longer, after having escaped the jaws of fatal heart attacks in our 60s, we often find ourselves slipping into dementia. Recent statistics show that dementia has overtaken heart disease as the leading cause of death in several parts of the Western world.

Slowing of the mind, slipping into dementia, and thereafter slithering into a coma is the next hazard. Its consequences can be challenging and devastating, not just to the patient but also to the family.

How does one look after a demented relative in these times? Our families are no longer the large undivided ones where there was always someone at home to care for them. We are now more often nuclear and sometimes even fragmented, living in towns and cities with all members rushing to work in the mornings and returning late just for dinner and sleep.

Reliance on domestic help is a threat and a luxury. Apart from security concerns, how sure can I be that the caregiver is not being harsh or cruel to my father during my absence? The patient may not even be able to remember or complain.

Institutional care is not an easy option. Apart from making most Indians feel guilty and with the high costs involved, most care centres are notorious for rough regimented jail-like treatment. The demented relative will of course flash a generous smile when you visit and not remember to tell you of what he had been put through, as he has lost his memory for recent things.

What is worrying about Alzheimer's disease, the typical and most common cause of dementia, is that we are making very little progress in finding a cure.

For instance, while there are close to 6,000 ongoing trials to discover cures for cancer, there are only 99 for Alzheimer's, laments Alice Thomson, a British researcher.

This empty space of medical therapy has, therefore, been filled by several claimants such as green tea, chocolates, fruits, nuts, green vegetables, and antioxidants, that are largely speculative.

But when you see your own parent going down the slippery slope of dementia, forgetting to switch off the fire in the kitchen, wandering off to an unknown area during an evening walk and not knowing how to return, or forgetting the name of his favourite grandson, your desperation will drive you to try almost anything that, not just doctors, but even neighbours advise. Anything that brings a ray of hope to bring his mind back!

06

Depression: The Dark Corner of Our Mind

I have depression. But I prefer to say, 'I battle depression' instead of 'I suffer' from it. Because when depression hits, I hit back. Battle on...

As a healthcare professional, I am getting increasingly concerned about reports suggesting that we are a depressed nation.

An article is doing the rounds which says that every sixth person in India is depressed. Further, the World Happiness Index published in March 2019 placed India in the 140th position, something that I found disconcerting.

The issue is critical as whatever else we do assumes meaning only if it brings a measure of happiness or satisfaction to our lives.

Depression is a persistent negative emotion of sadness or worthlessness or feeling of 'dried up from inside, without anything exciting to look forward to'. Before labelling someone as being depressed, there are a few caveats.

Life is bound to have its downturns, and a sense of grief or loss can engulf you, say at the bereavement of a dear one, a separation, or a loss in business. This grief is expected to run its course over a period of time.

When does grief become depression? If the emotion is too strong to make you contemplate taking drastic steps such as perhaps ending your own life, or if it runs too long such as spending the next year unable to come out and discharge other functions, such as looking after the children and family, it could be a matter of concern.

One form of depression is caused due to a trigger called 'reactive', which implies that it starts as a reaction to a life event. The other type is where there is a sense of 'drying up' without any identifiable cause. The patient often feels, "Everything is OK at home but I do not feel happy." This is called endogenous depression.

A simple 4-question screening test can help you recognise depression in yourself or in those around you (adapted from an article by Indu PS and colleagues):

Q1: Have you been experiencing sadness or are you in a depressed mood for the last two weeks or longer? Yes/No

Q2: Have you been experiencing a loss of interest or loss of pleasure in doing things in the last two weeks or longer? Yes/No

Q3: Have you been feeling excessively tired or without energy during the last two weeks or longer? Yes/No

Q4: Have you been suffering from sleeplessness, during the last two weeks or longer? Yes/No

If your answer is a 'Yes' to two or more questions, you could be depressed and hence should consider meeting up with a doctor, counsellor, or mature friend (could be your parent or spouse) and get out of the gloomy state.

So what did you find about yourself?

It is time we address this issue that affects our health and lives.

Section H

Special Patients, Population, and Conditions

Everybody is a genius. But if you judge a fish by its ability to climb a tree, it will live its whole life believing that it is stupid.

01

Dyslexia and a Different Form of Talent

I don't 'suffer' from dyslexia. I suffer from the ignorance of people who think they know what I can and cannot do.
– Erica Cook

If you meet someone who appears intelligent, has bright ideas, comes across as emotionally warm, and is often creative, but carries a poor school scorecard that had only tested his abilities to Read, Remember, Recall, and wRite, he could be a dyslexic. If you take a closer look at him, you may discover that he has a fantastic sense of colour, can paint well, picks up tunes and music much better than fellow students in his class, or has very creative ideas, often thinking out of the box. In fact, you could well be looking at a genius with tremendous potential.

Dyslexics, comprising five per cent of the population, can be spotted from a very young age. Typically, these kids have bright intelligent eyes, seem to follow what you tell them, react intelligently to situations, and are emotionally normal, but seem to get into problems when asked to read or write. They may sit with the book open for long hours without progressing down the page, write poorly with lots of spelling mistakes, confuse b with d (mirror images), and hence get poor marks in the way tests are 'normally' conducted.

They are certainly not mentally weak. In fact, studies show that some of the brightest and most successful have had the trait. Albert Einstein, the great scientist; John Lennon of Beatles fame; Richard Branson, the owner of Virgin Airlines; Tom Cruise, the Hollywood star; Thomas Edison, who gave us the electric bulb; Winston Churchill, the British PM are some examples of immensely successful people with dyslexia.

The problem with dyslexia is not with intelligence but with the wiring in the brain that deals with the way we learn or reproduce the symbols of language, such as alphabets or words, especially the written ones. Language, especially alphabets and words, have been made by man as an instrument for communication, and is, therefore, not something truly 'natural'. Dyslexics have a problem learning symbols of this man-made language and hence struggle in assessments that test the ability to learn and reproduce them.

What complicates the lives of dyslexic children is that parents as well as school teachers are often not aware or trained to pick up dyslexia. The trauma of a lovable bright child starts when he underperforms in his first written test, gets poor grades, and is told that he is dull or inattentive. Parents are then informed in PTMs that their child is mentally weak. Imagine how we would feel if we were told that we were dull just because we could not reproduce or write words or sentences well, but we had wonderful skills in painting, music, or designing that our teachers never tested us at!

That is the tragedy. Dyslexics are often very creative and artistic and can leave their 'scholar' colleagues way behind if only they were tested at what they were gifted with—art, design, music, creativity, etc. They would grow up and make the list of geniuses longer and brighter.

Amir Khan's Taare Zameen Par helped bring dyslexia to society's notice. Now special training modules are available that can help dyslexic children learn language well and rub shoulders with the toppers of his class. Picking these kids with special traits up at an early age, perhaps in preschool, is what we need to strive for. Our dyslexic geniuses will then realise their true potential and lead us forward with their creativity.

02

Blind Children Love Watching TV

The only thing worse than being blind is having sight but no vision. – Helen Keller

Children of Navjyoti School for the Blind, located in Mohanlalganj (in the city of Lucknow, India) love 'watching' serials on TV. "They follow the family dramas and all that is happening in the country by listening to the voices on TV and picturing the characters in their minds," says Sister Jessy, principal of the school that houses 65 blind children aged 6 to 14 years.

And if your eyes turn moist with sadness for these 'deprived' children, just hold on! They do not feel deprived as they do not know what they miss by way of vision, as they never had it. The term for them is neither deprived nor handicapped, but 'challenged', indicating that their inability to see poses a challenge for them to achieve almost all that their visually equipped colleagues can. They can sing, dance, play on the swings, study, pass exams, and get jobs. The way they appreciate beauty may, however, be somewhat different: Shreya Ghoshal may be more beautiful to them than Kareena Kapoor, as they perceive the world through voice and sounds.

I was amazed to see these children put up a group dance in which they came together, at times, with their out-stretched swinging hands meeting that of their partners in perfect harmony; so strong was their spatial sense that they could almost 'see' where the partner's hand was at that moment. They also put up a play where their lack of vision made no dent in how they moved around on the stage, faced each other, and acted their parts.

Suman showed me how she reads and writes without any vision. Her books and notes were in Braille, a form in which the paper is perforated or elevated in patterns so that alphabets and numbers can be recognised by touching them with her fingers. The school also has computers equipped with software that converts the alphabets that we recognise by their 2-dimensional shapes into Braille forms.

Blindness afflicts 1.5 per cent of our population making India the country with the largest number of blind people (15 million) of the globally estimated 37 million. Lack of vision in children may be of several types. Some can see at birth and then lose it due to damage to their corneas commonly caused by deficiency of vitamin A, or they may have very high refractive errors like myopia, while some may be blind from birth, as most children in this school are. They have perfectly normal intelligence and an enhanced sense of touch and sound.

The children of Navjyoti love music; they sing very well and are very fond of learning to play sitar and drums. And what touched me most was to see that they could laugh and play, and be happy, putting many long-faced people with 'sights' to shame. A visit to this school taught me much about life.

03

Lady Gaga Drags Fibromyalgia into the Spotlight

Pain that makes you want to walk away from your own body. My pain is invisible, and so is the pain you inflict when you don't believe me.

Limelight and controversies are not new to the international super-celebrity singer and star, Lady Gaga. I remember the first time I heard of her was when she had donned her famous nauseating meat dress to shock the world in her campaign against eating animal meat.

In keeping with the unusual campaigns that she seems to love doing, alongside her singing, she has recently started drawing the attention of the world to a relatively poorly understood medical condition, called fibromyalgia, which she is suffering from, and that has been interfering with her singing tours and career.

Fibromyalgia syndrome is a common and chronic disorder characterised by widespread pain, tenderness over most parts of the body when pressed, and tiredness. Typically the patient, usually a woman, complains of aches and muscle spasms or tightness over the limbs, bones, muscles, back, and head. The symptoms are distressing enough to interfere with normal life.

It is often associated with moderate to severe fatigue, decreased energy, insomnia, or waking up feeling just as tired as when you went to sleep.

Some report stiffness upon waking or after staying in one position for too long.

Patients with fibromyalgia also more often report symptoms of IBS, migraine, and dysmenorrhoea. Anxiety and depression are also common.

The real challenge is for the doctor to diagnose the condition, as there is no blood test to diagnose the condition. This limitation has resulted in the frequent inflicting of the label 'psychological' or 'all-in-the-head', which has worsened the fate of sufferers and stifled research into this condition.

Yes, low levels of vitamin D, and neuropathies due to conditions like diabetes and depression may co-exist, but fibromyalgia stands out as a distinct entity that persists despite correction of these factors.

What then makes the medical world believe that fibromyalgia is a distinct entity rather than a 'psychosomatic disorder' or a somatic expression of anxiety or depressive state?

Recent advances in functional imaging of the brain using FMRI have shown that these patients truly have a lowered threshold of body pain. Therefore, for the same amount of muscle stretching or squeezing that a normal person tolerates comfortably, these patients react with pain and spasms.

Scientists are still quite in the dark as to why there is this difference in response between normal persons and patients. Also, they are equally perplexed as to why these patients have increased frequency of other functional disorders such as migraine and IBS.

The answers may be still far, but Lady Gaga's attempt to drag this medical syndrome into the spotlight seems to have already generated considerable research interest into its causes, mechanisms, and treatment.

04

Parkinson's Disease: Muhammad Ali's Last Fight

Nothing lasts forever, that is the tragedy and miracle of existence. All we can do is make the best of the time we have. And go down shooting naturally. – Mira Grant

Muhammad Ali, one of the greatest sportsmen and legendary boxers of all time, died at the not-too-young age of 74, but his 30-year-long battle with the debilitating Parkinson's disease (PD) proved to be the most difficult fight of his life.

The features of Parkinson's disease are just the opposite of what the swift and agile Cassius Clay (his earlier name that he changed later to Muhammad Ali) stood for. It slows movements, makes the body stiff and rigid, and causes hands to shake with tremors. All these made Ali quite an antithesis of what he was earlier described as: 'floats like a butterfly and stings like a bee'.

Parkinson's disease is a degenerative condition of the brain that afflicts one in 100 people above age 60. Slowness of movement, rigidity of the body, and tremors of the hands characterise it. The gait becomes shuffling with small steps. A patient finds it hard to start walking, but once he starts, he shuffles along, sometimes finding it difficult to stop, change directions, or tackle steps and obstacles. The tremor of hands is quite characteristic and is described by doctors as a 'pill-rolling' movement. The handwriting becomes small, a feature called micrographia.

A difficult moment in Ali's life was the opening ceremony of the 1996 Olympics in Atlanta where he had to light the Olympic flame. Millions across the globe watched him take the torch in his violently shaking hands, and light the lamp with agonising slowness and difficulty. His face was also mask-like and his speech slow and slurred, all features of florid Parkinsonism.

The underlying mechanism of PD is the drying up of a neurotransmitter called dopamine from the lower regions of the brain called basal ganglia, that regulate body movement. Neurologists are still not clear what makes this chemical diminish in some.

There has been speculation that Muhammad Ali's Parkinsonism could have resulted from repeated trauma to the brain from innumerable head punches. He is reported to have received 440 blows in his deadliest last major fight with Joe Frasier three years before he hung up his gloves. Also striking is the fact that Ali developed PD two decades early.

Treatment is usually with medications that boost dopamine levels in the brain and reduce tremors and stiffness. Indian researchers claim that the household spice, turmeric, could help treat Parkinson's disease. It contains curcumin, a rich antioxidant, that scientists from IIIT-A and NIMHANS, Bangalore, feel could emerge as a useful remedy.

A positive aspect of Muhammad Ali's story for patients with PD is that it is possible to survive for 30 years with it, remaining clear in mind and doing much of what he wanted to do, despite physical limitations.

05

Alzheimer's Disease

Alzheimer's doesn't just steal memories, it steals identities and relationships.

The quick-witted and dashing trade union leader George Fernandes, went on to become the Defence Minister of India and is remembered for his fabled flight in a MIG fighter aircraft, but now unable to recognise his own relatives and recall his name. The 'cowboy' American President Ronald Reagan, the tough no-nonsense British prime minister Margaret Thatcher, and the Hollywood heartthrob Charlton Heston are among the 26 million people worldwide who are afflicted by Alzheimer's disease, which robs them of mental functions and reduces them to a blank vegetative state till death.

Alzheimer's disease (AD) is on the rise. The mother of a senior executive in Lucknow, who suffered from this disease and had become comatose, was, in a rare show of devotion, kept alive for five long years with life support at home. And some healthy relatives have cobbled together a group to learn and share about how to care for their affected seniors.

The disease starts usually after 65 and manifests slowly and subtly with forgetfulness of recent events and names (What did the new plumber say his name was? Who had come home last night to meet us?). Some may experience changes in moods, such as undue concern and anxiety, forgetting to do daily chores, the way back home from an evening walk, or failing to find the right words during conversations. The withdrawal then begins, as the person sinks into apathy (not quite bothered about a family function going on in the drawing room) and the stare becomes blank and hollow.

The burden of AD on the family can be heavy. When a husband fails to recognise his spouse of 40 years, it can shatter hearts. Relatives are often caught in a dilemma of whether to let life go on, with the affected senior confined to a room with hired attendants (often bringing feelings of guilt), or cut out much of the fun of life and stay together indoors with the patient (not fair to young children, but it often hardly matters to the patient as he is obtunded and apathetic).

What causes AD is unclear and is the subject of intense global research. The brain shrinks and develops plaques of a jelly-like substance called amyloid. One of the chemical transmitters of the brain, acetylcholine, dries up leading to poor functioning and networking between various parts of the brain.

While the quest for a magic potion for AD continues, scientists have been trying to identify who might be at risk (smokers, diabetics, hypertensives) and what factors might prevent one from suffering from it (high consumption of fresh fruits, chocolates, coffee, and interest in board games). The familiar dietary ingredient, haldi (turmeric, curcumin), loaded with antioxidants, has emerged as a front-runner for the cure.

When I see a patient with AD I am reminded of the old adage, *All good things in life are lent, not given.* Our fertile brains are no exception!

06

Ageing

Life humbles you as you age. You realise how much time you wasted on nonsense.

As an increasing number of people in developed countries are living longer with the elderly comprising a significant proportion of the population, the best brains and laboratories are researching as to why we grow old. Divisions are sometimes made between the young old (65–74), the middle old (75–84), and the oldest old (85+). However, chronological age does not correlate well with functional age, i.e., two people may be of the same age but differ in their mental and physical capacities—some people at 85 may play golf and be mentally alert, while another person at 65 may be bedridden with diabetes, stroke, and dementia.

The term 'ageing' is somewhat ambiguous, but refers to the physical, psychological, and social changes that occur as one grows in years. Some dimensions of ageing grow and expand over time, while others decline. Reaction time, for example, may slow with age, while knowledge of world events and wisdom may expand which explains why the proportion of elderly among politicians tends to be high. Research shows that even late in life, there still is potential for physical, mental, and social growth and development.

What causes the body, with all its organs and tissues, to grow old? Why does the skin wrinkle, hair turn grey, and the list of diseases like diabetes, blood pressure, cataracts, and heart problems grow long? Why do we start slowing down, and also why do we become prone to a variety of cancers? The process seems to start with the cells in our body showing signs of ageing, called senescence, which occurs due to the progressive shortening of one of its parts called the telomere. The cell dies each time the cell divides when the telomere becomes too short. The length of telomeres is, therefore, the 'molecular clock', and what maintains the telomere length is an enzyme called telomerase.

Why then does the telomere shorten quickly in some, and how can we keep our telomerase enzyme levels high? In 2007, researchers at the Salk Institute for Biological Studies identified a critical gene that specifically links eating fewer calories with living longer and showed that the gene pha-4 regulates the longevity response to CRs. Semi-starved rats live much longer compared to well-fed ones, and slim beauty winners may actually live longer than their wholesome counterparts.

Apart from the role of longevity determining genes (LDG), cumulative tissue stress arising from the release of oxygen radicals during cell metabolism has been another suspect. Ageing tissues are deficient in antioxidants such as tocopherol, ascorbic acid, and retinol that are normally found in fresh fruits and vegetables; hence the recommendation of five helpings of such food items every day. Whether the synthetic antioxidants sold as capsules do any good to keep our tissues young is yet to be proven.

Researchers have now identified compounds that can actually increase telomerase levels, and thereby stop the ageing process. Resveratrol, Rapamycin, acetyl-L-carnitine, and alpha-lipoic acid are currently undergoing research.

As the quest for eternal youth continues, the two ancient Parijaat trees standing majestically in Barabanki and Sultanpur, which are fabled to have provided agelessness to our gods and goddesses, could hold the secret!

07

Palliative Care: Adding Life to Days

How you make others feel says a lot about who you are.
Leave them with a smile, a hug, and a kind thought.

While medical science has significantly increased our life expectancy and made many diseases treatable, it has made our expectations soar to unreasonable heights and diminished our capacity to accept death due to diseases that defy current treatment. Widespread cancer, dementia, and advanced chronic diseases of the heart, lungs, or liver are some examples that cause significant pain and suffering, progress relentlessly, and render even relatives helpless and frustrated.

Palliative Medicine (PM) may sound like a paradox in modern times, as "it aims to add life or quality to the remaining days in terminally ill patients," said Dr. Mhoira Leng, a British doctor presently working in Uganda, and a pioneer in this subspeciality, when she was in Lucknow. "Providing relief from the distressing and dehumanising pain to patients with terminal cancer can be one of the greatest boons of medical science that is unfortunately not often adequately utilised," she added.

Experts in PM have to tackle several problems at various stages. Their work often starts with breaking the bad news and counselling such patients and relatives, who are often in a state of denial or unrealistic expectations. Relatives of most cancer patients in India do not wish the diagnosis to be disclosed to the patient. As the disease progresses and hospital visits get more frequent, the patient usually starts suspecting the diagnosis but finds himself surrounded by bluffing relatives, with whom he can no longer discuss with frankness his problems, preferences, and last wishes. He often feels lonely and emotionally isolated in his last days.

At stake is the care that such patients receive. To most relatives (read well-earning sons often staying elsewhere), it means taking the ailing parent from one hospital to another, often to another city, putting them through a battery of expensive re-tests, and hooking him on to machines in ICU setups, and keeping them ignorant of their diagnosis and fate. While all this provides some satisfaction to the relatives that they have done all that they possibly could, and mitigates their sense of guilt, it often adds to the patients' misery, pain, and suffering. Studies have shown that what they need most is their own bed, their familiar home, loving relatives, and palliation of distressing symptoms that make the agonising last phase of life bearable.

Relief of pain is crucial to caring for such patients. A recent study has shown that specialists in tertiary care hospitals are often more obsessed with performing one test after another and paying much less importance to relieve pain. The recently started Pain Clinic and the PM services at SGPGI hope to change that. After assessing the severity of pain, therapy is tailored to the patient's requirement. Apart from providing relief to the distressed patient and making him comfortable, it often soothes the nerves of bewildered relatives. The major challenge is to take such therapy to the patient's bedside at home.

Jade Goody, the British TV star, died recently of advanced cervical cancer. Rather than in an alien atmosphere of a hospital surrounded by machines, she lived her last days with dignity at home, and that is where she preferred to die.

08

Euthanasia: Compassion or Crime?

It seems most strange to me that men should fear, that death is a necessary end, and will come when it will come.
– William Shakespeare

Lazer, the pet dog who had reached a ripe old age of 15 had become blind, bedridden, and pitiful from constant pain from many age-related ailments, and had begun to weigh heavily on the hearts of the Mithals. Unable to see him in constant agony anymore, they decided to put him to sleep as a final act of compassion.

Vibhav (name changed), who is now taking up a job after completing law school recalled how Lazer had entered their home and hearts as a tender one-month-old pup when he was in second standard. Over 16 years, Lazer had played several roles from being the youngest child to Ranjana and Ambrish to a younger brother, playmate, friend, and guard to Varun and Vibhav.

Lazer had brought that special mirth and cheerfulness to their home: playfully teasing the children out of bed by pulling off their sheets, naughtily hiding their socks when they were getting ready for school, guarding their home all day, welcoming them back with incessant wagging of his tail, and playing ball with them in the evenings.

But as one year of a dog's life is equivalent to seven of a man's, Lazer fast-tracked from a baby to youth to mid-life to senility in 16 years (equivalent to 112 of a man) with cataract, diabetes, weak heart, and paralytic legs, as he lay immobile and groaned constantly in pain. After much deliberation, he was released from his painful state by euthanasia or mercy killing.

While most animal lovers would approve of mercy killing for suffering animals, extrapolating a similar approach to humans never fails to stir the hornet's nest.

Counterarguments usually begin with our arrogant positioning that *Man is not an animal*! While there certainly are differences, the similarities of the cycle of life and death are inescapably similar and humbling. Any person who has lived with and seen an elderly relative struck with an incurable progressive disease like cancer, wither and groan to the predictable painful end, will testify having wished an early respite for their loved ones.

Opposition to Euthanasia comes from both religious and legal quarters. The faithful argue that since man is incapable of creating life, how can he assume the right to snuff it out? Some go further to explain that the misery needs to be suffered through as it is ordained.

On the legal and technical fronts, there are three major concerns: How sure can we be that the situation is truly irretrievable? How can we be sure that this is what the suffering person, who is presently comatose, would have wanted? And lastly, with sanctioning to (mercy) kill, what is the possibility for ingenuous humans to misuse it for selfish gains?

The Mithals heaved a sigh of relief on letting suffering Lazer go, preferring to keep the memories of his younger frolicking days in their hearts. And as we remain uncertain about how to deal with humans in similar situations, we keep doing what we are best at—procrastinating.

Section I

Medical Emergencies

An accident won't arrive with a bell on its neck
– Finnish proverb

01

Peanuts: The Biggest Choking Hazard

If you close your eyes to facts, you will learn through accidents.
– African Proverb

It is hard to imagine that the small unassuming ubiquitous peanut, that we love to munch, could be most hazardous for infants, toddlers, and preschool children.

I recently heard the story of a toddler who choked while eating peanuts and died a couple of days later after a traumatic and tragic course.

That morning was like any other with a session of peanut-munching at home with his sibs, when this two-year-old suddenly choked, started coughing, and became breathless. His parents rushed him to a nearby hospital where x-rays and scans showed a 'nut' stuck and obstructing the windpipe near its bifurcation in the chest.

He was then shifted to a centre that had facilities for bronchoscopy, a procedure that involves passing a type of endoscope into the windpipe, to remove the nut.

As one can imagine, all this took a while, and by the time the procedure could be done, it was midnight. The child's respiration and blood pressure fell during attempts to catch the nut that was by now, stuck in the bronchus. As bad luck would have it, the nut continued wedging its way further down, defying all attempts at catching it. The child's condition deteriorated finally ending in death.

The catapulting of a happy family with a toddling bundle of joy to one of death and gloom, caused by a peanut could not have been more sardonic. I was reminded of the jolt we had felt 30 years ago on hearing how our friend's baby had choked and died on his first birthday that was being celebrated in the USA.

Experience from across the world tells us that peanuts are the most common cause of death due to aspiration in small kids. It is followed by other nuts, marshmallows, carrots, and candies.

Small kids like to explore the world by constantly putting anything they can get their tiny hands on, into their mouths.

As a gastroenterologist, we get our share of ingested 'foreign bodies' stuck in the food pipe of kids. Two months ago, while I was having dinner at a restaurant with visiting guests, I got an emergency call to retrieve a coin from the food pipe of a three-year-old. That day had been fortunately easy and lucky for all of us.

Coming back to the question: Why are nuts the most common items on which kids choke? Well, nuts are hard and need to be chewed and crushed before swallowing—acts that require using molar teeth located at the back of the jaw. It turns out that molars start appearing after three years of age. Therefore, we should not get misguided by the toothy smiles of kids. They reveal the front teeth comprising incisors and canines that can bite and cut, but not chew.

It is a gruesome reminder: Do not keep nuts and carrots on the table if you have toddlers at home and let young parents you can reach out to know this.

02

Severe Allergic Reactions

Springtime is like a box of tissues – full of sneezes and allergies. My favourite springtime fashion accessories are antihistamines.
– Anon

The range of allergies can be huge, from a simple sneeze or an occasional itch to angry hives, asthma, breathlessness, and shock. An allergic reaction often comes on at odd times without warning and in funny places far from access to medical help.

I strongly recommend each one of you to read the true story of a young girl in Ireland, so that you never find yourself in such a trap.

'Mother's agony as teenage girl dies from peanut allergy on city street

This is the tragic story of teenager Emma Sloan who died on a city street just minutes after suffering a fatal allergic reaction. Emma (14) was out for a pre-Christmas meal with her family when she accidentally ate a nut-based sauce and suffered a severe allergic reaction.

But when her mother rushed to a nearby pharmacy to get help, she was refused a lifesaving adrenaline injection because she didn't have a prescription.

The distraught mother was told to bring her daughter to hospital but the two had only got a few yards away when the teenager collapsed.

Emma's mother, Caroline, told the Irish Independent: "I'm so angry, I was not given the EpiPen to inject her. I was told to bring Emma to an A&E department.

My daughter died on a street corner with a crowd around her. How could a peanut kill my child?

Emma has always been very careful and would check the ingredients of every chocolate bar and other foods to be sure they didn't contain nuts," her mother Caroline said.

"I'm not blaming the restaurant because there was a sign saying 'contains nuts' but it wasn't noticed. After a while, Emma began to say, 'I can't breathe, I can't breathe'.

He told me, I couldn't get it without a prescription. He told me to bring her to A&E.

I left and I knew we'd have to run all the way to Temple Street hospital. But she only got as far as the corner of Abbey Street when she collapsed. She died on the footpath," said the grieving mother, fighting back tears.

"A doctor was passing and had tried to help and put her into the recovery position. Ambulance and fire brigade men worked on her. But she was gone."

Allan O'Keefe, The Independent, December 20, 2013', abridged.

Yes, sudden allergic reactions can be serious and sometimes fatal and claim 3,000 lives each year in the USA. And your doctor can be of little help if you come down with it while you are having dinner at a far-off destination.

I, therefore, recommend carrying anti-allergy tablets with you in your purse or bag at all times: a tablet of Avil, Allegra, Cetrizine, Alspan, or some such for mild ones, and two tablets of Prednisolone (steroid) for serious ones. Adrenaline injection remains the life-saver for the very serious types that the young girl suffered.

While we Indians have been rapped too often for allowing easy access to medicines, I wonder if the rigidity of the Irish rules cost Emma her life.

03

Medical Strangulation

If someone grabbed me, I'd probably be able to choke them out in about eight seconds. – Jeffrey Donovan

Gayatri (name changed), a 31-year-old pretty vivacious woman who works as a medical administrator in a corporate hospital and stays alone in an apartment, has been perpetually frightened ever since she survived a near-death experience from suffocation a year ago.

Over the last two years, every now and then, she suddenly breaks out into angry itchy hives all over her body, along with a feeling of choking that makes her gasp for breath.

She recounts in horror when she had a bad attack one early morning while she was alone at home. Soon after, the skin hives started appearing, and she felt as though someone was tightening a noose around her throat. She gradually turned blue and lost consciousness.

Luckily, she was able to pick up her cell phone and make a call to her doctor-friend who, sensing something seriously wrong rushed to her home and injected her with adrenaline, which saved her in the nick of time.

Subsequent tests showed that she suffered from a rare condition called angioedema, in which an individual is prone to develop swelling (or oedema) of the soft tissues and mucous membranes of the body on provocation by certain foods, medicines, bee stings, wasp bites, or minor trauma. When the swelling occurs in the neck, especially around the windpipe, it obstructs the air passages, sometimes causing death from suffocation.

Angioedema is rare, but many probably die due to a lack of recognition and timely action. Gayatri was fortunate as she worked in a hospital, and her caring medical colleagues were able to put her through the requisite tests and prove that she indeed has a deficiency of a C1 q esterase enzyme that is the hallmark of this condition.

Medical suffocation, be it from angioedema or anaphylaxis, a severe form of allergy, requires prompt recognition and action. Though intravenous injections of anti-allergics and corticosteroids often work, the specific therapy to turn things around is a subcutaneous injection of adrenaline.

A special pre-loaded adrenaline pen, or EpiPen as it is called, looks quite like an insulin pen, and is easy to self-use. It has helped save many lives. One just needs to jab it on one's thigh and inject it.

That delay can cost lives was realised when a 14-year-old Irish girl, Emma Sloan died of peanut allergy in a restaurant a few years ago. Seeing her daughter get breathless in a restaurant, her mother had rushed to the nearby chemist's shop to procure an EpiPen. The Irish chemist refused to dispense the injection without a valid medical prescription. The young girl had collapsed and died minutes later.

Saving lives is sometimes all about timing and promptness. In the words of JFK, "The difference between salad and garbage is in the timing."

My naughty mind often wonders what would be the fate of such patients if our courts were to decide on their treatment.

04

Sudden Cardiac Arrest - CPR (Cardio-Pulmonary Resuscitation)

In every moment, you have the power to hit the reset button and start anew.

Can you do cardiac resuscitation?

If you were to see a person 'drop dead' all of a sudden, are you capable of doing the hands-on cardiac resuscitation?

Here are some facts for you:

- Every year in India, around 700, 000 (7 lac) people have sudden cardiac arrest (SCA) where the heart suddenly stops beating and pumping blood to organs, leading to sudden death.
- Around a third are aged under 50.
- What makes the difference between dying and coming back to life for a person who develops SCA is a timely revival with CPR.
- Calling an ambulance or a doctor is what we all do, but by the time they arrive (after over 15 minutes or more, in many countries), the organs of the body would have undergone irreversible damage. Hence many are declared to be 'brought dead' by the time they reach the hospital. Timely CPR while waiting for help is ESSENTIAL.
- Most cardiac arrests occur at home; some in place of work or in public places. It could happen to someone close to you too.

SCA made a dramatic re-entry into the public mind when,

Damar Hamlin, a 34-year-old celebrated American football player, suddenly collapsed on the ground during a match, to the horror of spectators. It took just a couple of minutes to realise that he had sustained an SCA. His heart had stopped beating, and he was almost dead.

Paramedics then rushed to the field and started thumping Hamlin's chest, giving him an external cardiac massage. He was resuscitated within nine minutes, restarting the stopped heart, just in time to save his brain from damage. He was then shifted to hospital where he was treated further and is now back home.

The American Cardiac Association acknowledges and stresses how TIMELY action (mind you, not the BEST, by a famous cardiologist) can save more lives, and reinforces the need for banking on paramedics and 'common' people to provide it.

Several movements are already on to provide training and make every person 'CPR literate' as one never knows when the situation could arise.

Individuals in institutions such as schools, colleges, and offices, and transport crews are particularly encouraged to learn first aid and CPR.

Remember, it could happen in your home too; many of us live years cursing doctors and hospitals for someone we lost but shrink away from the uncomfortable question, "Could you have done things differently?"

Learn about CPR by reading up on Damar Hamlin's story and join in on a CPR training course.

05

Good old Aspirin for Cardiac Emergency

Most things in this world don't work, aspirin does.
– Kurt Vonnegut

Heart attacks are common above 40, often coming at odd times, without warning, and are the most common killer of our modern times. The best chances of reducing the severity of an acute attack and improving the chances of survival are by chewing aspirin at the very start and reaching a hospital within two hours.

A doctor colleague of mine, Dr. Anil Behl, has started a unique form of social service, of putting four aspirin tablets in a plastic pouch and keeping it available at all times with the security check-post of his housing colony. He has backed up this simple act by informing all residents of his colony by email and posters, that should anyone have early symptoms of heart attack, they should immediately procure the pills from the security room and chew them while waiting for further help to arrive.

During a heart attack, blood clot forms in the arteries of the heart blocking the flow of oxygen-rich blood to heart muscles. Clot formation begins with the clumping of small blood particles called platelets. What aspirin does is that it prevents stickiness and clumping of platelets. When taken during a heart attack it slows clotting and decreases the size of the clot.

Most cardiologists swear by aspirin for several reasons.

For those who have had a heart attack previously, long-term use of aspirin reduces the chances of having a second one. It is useful for those who have never had a heart disease before but are at increased risk of having one. This group includes people above 40 who have diabetes, high blood pressure, increased levels of cholesterol, and smokers. Those with a strong family history of heart disease also come in the 'risky' category.

A daily dose of low-dose aspirin has been shown to reduce the risk of a first heart attack in this group. Cardiologists also recommend aspirin to all those who have had a cardiac artery bypass surgery or angioplasty. The reasons are much the same. It prevents platelets from clumping thus reducing the chances of clot formation in the arteries of the heart.

Heart attack presents as heaviness or pain in the centre of the chest, often radiating to the neck, left arm, or back, sometimes associated with sweating and uneasiness. It is often felt as gas and vomiting by some.

Section J

Other Medical Topics

Never regret anything that has happened in your life.
It cannot be changed, undone or forgotten, so take it as a
lesson learned and move on.

01

TB Is Invading Our Homes

When TB knocks on the door of our homes, let unity, knowledge and compassion be our strongest defences.

When Mr. Randeep (name changed), a 55-year-old industrialist and politician, who came to see me for crampy abdominal pain and weight loss over six months, was detected to have an ulcer in the intestine due to tuberculosis, he reacted with shock and disbelief. To him, tuberculosis (TB) was an infection that happened to 'others' in slums and villages.

With 2.6 million Indians estimated to be suffering from TB, we account for one in every five across the world. And with 3.87 lakh people acquiring the infection every year, India is emerging as an epidemic bed of TB, claiming a life every two minutes.

The disease is now invading our homes, with people from the middle and upper classes no longer being able to remain immune to it. In fact, a large number of people coming to me from well-off homes with the infection are surprised at how they contracted it.

The infection gets into our body through the air we breathe. The germ, mycobacterium tuberculosis, spreads through droplets that a person with TB of the lungs coughs or spits, and sprays into the air. Further, once coughed out, the germ tends to hover around in the air for long periods, allowing us to inhale them unknowingly.

Most infections, therefore, occur in public places: buses, metros, trains, railway stations, crowded classes, and offices. Family members of an infected person are more likely to inhale droplets at home, the chances increase with crowding and poor ventilation.

Tuberculosis of the lungs is easily diagnosed in a person who has been coughing for over a month, running a low-grade temperature, especially in the evenings, and losing weight. A chest x-ray and sputum test can help confirm the same.

The problem, however, is that most patients do not necessarily present in this classical manner. A person may be running low-grade fever for weeks and losing weight for instance, but his chest x-ray may be normal, a situation that happens with infection of other organs. How does one diagnose extra-pulmonary TB?

Blood tests for diagnosis of TB, such as ELISA, are extremely unreliable and have, therefore, been banned by the government. A skin test called PPD tells about a past exposure to the germ that most of us have had and does not tell about an active disease. Scans such as ultrasound or CT scans may show glands and shadows but do not tell their nature, adding to the diagnostic challenges faced by the clinician.

Another cause for concern is that the germ is showing resistance to commonly used drugs. In fact, it has metamorphosed from being resistant to a single drug to MDR (multi-drug resistance), and now to one called TDR (total drug resistance), posing a major threat to all of us.

The germ that was discovered by Robert Koch in 1882 has indeed given mankind a long run and does not seem to be in a relenting mood in coming times either. Tuberculosis germ is indeed lurking around.

02

NOCEBO Effect: Expecting Adverse Effects of Medications Often Help Create Them

Just as positive thoughts can heal, negative thoughts can harm. The NOCEBO effect is a testament to the power of the mind.

Funny as it might seem, patients who are warned too much of possible side effects before being given a medication, seem to experience them more often. Describing this phenomenon as the NOCEBO effect, German researcher, Winfried Hauser, has recently shown that patients anticipating side effects such as giddiness, headache, constipation, or lack of concentration, experience them more often than those who take the drug without being told about them.

This new finding fits well with what physicians have suspected all along, that the body's response to therapy often depends on the patient's belief with which he takes it. Some of the benefits of medicine undoubtedly come from the positive anticipation that a particular drug will work as intended—easing arthritis or relieving wheezing, for example—called the PLACEBO effect. On the flip side, our belief in a drug's side effects may actually cause us to suffer from them as well.

The role of suggestion and belief in obtaining a positive response from treatment is well known. Scientists have shown that PLACEBO medication, one which has no active ingredient but looks like a drug, such as an empty capsule, often produces remarkable benefits when taken with positive anticipation of relief. As many as 50 per cent of patients report benefits in headaches, abdominal pain, dyspepsia, and sexual dysfunctions with dummy medicines consumed in good faith.

Dr. Winfried Hauser, a German expert in psychosomatic medicine, who has visited India two times, feels that the imagination and fears of patients can have just the opposite effect. When cautioned that a drug may cause sexual dysfunction, for example, a larger number of patients taking it report experiencing it.

A lady who consulted me with a history of breaking into allergic hives on taking virtually every antibiotic had a similar reaction when administered a vitamin capsule that looked like an antibiotic. Her hives disappeared when she was told and assured that it was a vitamin and not an antibiotic.

Practitioners of alternative and indigenous systems of medicine bank more on faith and do not usually mention the side effects of their therapy. Patients too, therefore, consider these innocuous and harmless, and consequently do not report side effects with their use.

Is keeping patients in the dark about a drug's potential side effects, then the only solution? In modern times it would be clearly not ethical. What experts propose is 'contextualised informed consent' that takes into account the possible side effects, the patient being treated, and the disease involved. While it will be clearly important to caution against potentially dangerous side effects, such as drowsiness while prescribing anti-allergic drugs to a person who might drive a car for instance, mentioning lack of concentration with an anti-diarrheal to an exam-going student may cause unnecessary harm.

Modern medicine, practiced with great caution and with a very defensive attitude as is done in litigant societies, requires that all potential effects of therapy, beneficial as well as harmful, be placed on the table. Which one to highlight and which ones to downplay remains somewhat subjective and a matter of the wise doctor's discretion.

03

Incidentaloma: Does all the Report Says Really Matter?

In the world of medical imaging, an incidentaloma can turn a routine scan into a life-altering moment.

The premise on which health checks are advised for a person who 'feels' normal, is that it may help pick up 'early' disease, that may be easier to manage, providing a longer and healthier life.

They do pick up quite a few health problems, which if addressed early, can make a positive impact on life. One, that is most convincing, is the detection of hypertension, or high blood pressure. Numerous studies have shown that if the high BP is controlled, it brings down the risk of heart disease, stroke, and renal disease significantly, and extends life expectancy. The same can be said of high blood sugar or diabetes.

The list is indeed long with thyroid disorders, heart problems, fatty liver, and high blood lipids, all squeezing themselves to join into the list.

One test that, however, proves to be double-edged, is the abdominal ultrasound. Data shows that around five per cent (in India) to 15 per cent (in the West) of people will discover that they have gallbladder stones and around 7 per cent (in India) will get to know that they have kidney stones. These have obviously formed quite a while ago but had been lying silent. Their discovery now drops the question: What needs to be done for them? Surgery?

It also picks up a large number of other problems that the person was unaware of till then. They have acquired the term incidentaloma as they are picked up incidentally. Around 20 per cent of adults harbour cysts in their kidneys or liver. These are innocuous and need not be approached as a disease, but once you come to know of them, the mind does go to the site where the ultrasound probe says the cyst is located.

Other common findings in the liver include hemangiomas, adenomas, old scars from previous infections, and some benign tumours. These 'discoveries' pose a new challenge, often prompting another set of detailed testing, to finally resolve matters. What goes on in the meantime is a good bit of uneasiness and worry in the patient's mind.

A senior doctor, who has become a good friend subsequently, had such a harrowing experience when he reluctantly underwent a routine checkup in 2015. Ultrasound examination showed a small tumour in the liver that had not caused him any symptoms. This finding led to a series of advanced tests such as a CT scan and MRI that confirmed that it was liver cancer. And there was not one, but three of them!

Several experts agreed with the interpretation of scan findings and diagnosis. By way of treatment, advice ranged from getting the liver transplanted (he is 71 now) to getting drugs injected into the tumour repeatedly to destroy as many of the tumour cells as possible in the hope of controlling or slowing the disease.

Unexpected discoveries are like the proverbial glass of water: Pessimists and anxious people see it as half-empty, finding it difficult to reconcile new information about disease and health. Optimists, however, would see the glass as half full.

04

Ruby's Food Pipe

In the darkness of corrosive injury, the human spirit shines brightest as survivors find strength they never knew they had.

Ruby finally underwent surgery for a blocked and ulcerated food pipe that had plagued her for 12 long years. This 30-year-old frail girl of 40 kilos got a second chance to live life with grace and vigour when a loop of intestine replaced her gullet and allowed her to eat normal food.

Her problems had begun suddenly 12 years prior to her visiting us when she had accidentally swallowed sulphuric acid used commonly as a floor cleaner in India, that her father had kept in a clear water bottle at home. She still shudders to think of the intense burning, pain, choking, and swelling around her mouth, and the agony of intravenous drips she required in the hospital. A week later she noticed difficulty in swallowing food that had progressed over weeks to a state when she could not swallow even her saliva. She had withered rapidly from a 55 kg energetic girl to a skin-and-bony 30 kg in three months. She had become so weak that she needed hospitalisation and intravenous drips periodically.

She had come to us at that stage with a badly strictured (narrowed) food pipe through which even water could not trickle down easily. We had managed to pass a thin wire across using an endoscope and dilate the stricture with bougies and balloons. This allowed liquids, and then, after a few more sessions, semi-solids such as sooji, khichri, and custards to pass down into her stomach. She soon picked up a few kilos and got back onto her feet.

Then the socio-economic factors came into play. Her parents found her protracted illness too expensive and decided to concentrate on their two other children, leaving Ruby to her fate. Her marriage of a few months broke up. She soon found herself struggling to stay alive, earning Rs 3,000 per month from a lodge as a part-time caretaker, and spending most of it on her two weekly dilatation sessions and her special liquid feeds.

She had been advised of surgery several times over this period but had declined. First, there was the issue of expense. Second, no family support. And third, she was mortally scared of losing her voice as she had met someone who had after this kind of surgery.

What then triggered this change of mind now? With her indomitable spirit, she had enrolled for a graduation course that she was pursuing after the day's work. Further, a benevolent soul, touched by her story, had offered to sponsor her surgery. She, on her part, had finally decided to take the risk and turn the corner. Her ambition then was to leave the unpleasant past behind, create her own future, and become independent.

Corrosive injury to the food pipe is still a common problem in India. While some are due to accidents, many occur from suicidal intent in a fit of desperation. Most victims are able to live normal lives with few sessions of endoscopic dilatation, but some like Ruby needed more help.

The surgery fortunately went off well. A portion of her large intestine was used to create a new tube connecting her upper portion of the food pipe to the stomach, bypassing her damaged narrowed oesophagus.

Though her recovery took a while longer because of her frail condition, she bounced back to health and gained weight.

After earning some money, she got married again. A year later she gave birth to a daughter, and now she is doing well in life in every way!

05

Acid Suppressants and Dementia

In medicine, as in life, every action has a reaction. The acid suppressant-dash debate reminds us to weigh the potential risks and benefits of our choices.

Your enemy, as they say, could well be sleeping in your backyard, especially when it comes to medications that have earned your trust and that you use frequently.

A group of medical scientists have rung alarm bells for the common acid suppressants called proton pump inhibitors, due to their association with dementia and heart attacks in elderly people who have been taking them for several years.

They noted that elderly people who had consumed PPIs for several years had dementia more often than those of similar age who had not taken them.

PPIs are commonly used for relieving burning in the chest (heartburn) or upper abdomen caused by gastric acid. The names of this group of drugs end with 'zole' such as omeprazole, esomeprazole, pantoprazole, or rabeprazole. They are the most effective medicines for treating acid-related symptoms, and due to their presumed safety profile, have become favourites with doctors and patients.

Their possible role in causing dementia found two tracks of explanation. PPI consumers often develop a deficiency of vitamin B12 or cyano-cobalamine, as this vitamin requires acid for absorption from the gut. Vitamin B12 plays a pivotal role in keeping our brains and nerves healthy. Deficiency of vitamin B12 is known to impair cognitive function, alertness, and memory.

The other concern has come from experimental observation in rats in which the brains of animals that were fed high doses of PPI were found to be filled with a rubbery amyloid-like substance that looks similar to the brains of humans with Alzheimer's disease.

On a similar note, Chinese doctors have reported a similar statistical association between elderly people taking PPIs and the frequency of heart attacks.

The risk of adverse effects of PPI, if they exist at all, is small, to the tune of one in 4,000 people who take these drugs regularly.

Authorities are still unsure whether this association suggests a causative role. However, with our life expectancy getting stretched and the number of red flags going up, notes of caution have started appearing in medical journals urging doctors to reduce unnecessary prescriptions of these drugs, especially for long periods.

Public opinion and sentiments have the habit of swinging like a pendulum from one extreme to another. To be fair to PPIs, let us not overlook the huge benefits they have brought to patients and the community. Peptic ulcers, especially the duodenal variety, used to be very frequent in the 70s when a large number of people suffered much, and many had to undergo surgery for duodenal narrowing or bleeding. Deaths due to ulcer disease that was quite common then, hardly occur nowadays, thanks to PPIs.

If you are hooked to PPIs, it is perhaps time, however, to explore alternate ways to keep your stomach and food pipe cool. Stepping down to H2RAs (ranitidine or famotidine) and soothing gels or antacid tablets may be a good idea after all.

06

Pain Killers Can Turn Killers

The irony of painkillers is that they can become life-takers when they lead to dependency and destruction.

The shocking death of the pop icon Michael Jackson at just 52 years, has drawn attention to the dangers of painkillers. The autopsy report ruled out blockage of the arteries of his heart and pointed to the consumption of excess amounts of painkillers and other medications as the cause of his collapse. Reports suggest that he was on to as many as seven drugs, comprising painkillers, muscle relaxants, and anti-depressants that made a deadly cocktail.

Pain killers or analgesics, are of two broad groups:

- Narcotic: such as morphine, extracted from opium, a product of the Poppy plant or its cousins, such as pethidine (Demerol*), hydromorphone (Dilaudid*, considered eight times more potent than pethidine), codeine (Vicodine*), oxycodone, tramadol, pentazocine, and others. These are strong analgesics used for severe pain and have potentially serious side effects such as drowsiness, coma, respiratory failure, circulatory failure, shock, and heart failure, apart from the strong potential for addiction and dependence. Many, such as pethidine, can be taken only as injections.
- Non-narcotic: such as paracetamol (as in Crocin or Tylenol), aspirin, ibuprofen (as in Brufen), piroxicam (as in Pirox), and

nimesulide (withdrawn from most countries). The most common problem with these drugs is irritation and bleeding from the stomach. They can also affect the liver and kidneys, but are not addictive and do not suppress breathing.

Apart from these side effects, painkillers can cross-react with each other as well as with a large number of other medications. Hence 'cocktails' are hazardous, as was with MJ.

In addition, MJ was on alprazolam (a sleeping pill as in Alprax, Trika, etc.), chlorpheniramine (anti-allergic, that can also cause drowsiness), and on two anti-depressants—sertraline (as in Serta, Daxid) and paroxetine (Paxil), that added to the toxicity. What probably precipitated his collapse was an injection of propofol, a drug that is used for general anaesthesia. It causes total loss of consciousness and depresses breathing, and hence is supposed to be used only by anaesthetists in a hospital setting where artificial ventilatory support is available.

Most narcotic analgesics are not available 'over the counter'. How MJ had access to three of them (marked*) is not clear. What is most intriguing is how he managed to get his doctor to administer an intravenous dose of propofol, at his home.

Irrational decisions are often made by a depressed and confused mind. MJ was undoubtedly suffering from depression and anxiety for which he was on medications. His financial losses and loneliness must have added to his frustration. He was probably addicted to narcotics for quite some time, as several injection marks on his body suggested. While the electrifying music of this musical genius will live on for many years, the story of his death should alert and remind us of the hazards of the indiscriminate use of painkillers.

07

Medical Accidents

Medical accidents remind us that while medicine is a science, it is also an art and each patient's case is unique.

If the thought of visiting a hospital makes butterflies flutter in your stomach, you are neither alone nor is the fluttering without cause. Hospitals are accident-prone zones, and often the news or memory of an adverse experience someone has had while in hospital might be the cause for your unconscious anxiety.

The WHO estimates that an accident might be occurring in as many as one in three hundred patients admitted to hospital, ranking tenth among the causes of hospital deaths. It accounts for approximately 30,000 deaths in the USA alone. Compare this with one in a million (1,000,000), the rate of accidents that occur in the airline industry, presently considered one of the safest.

Don't get me wrong and start imagining that hospitals gobble up a large number of healthy lives of cheerful people going on a holiday. In most instances, these are critically sick people on the proverbial razor's edge, who often tumble downhill after an intervention that retrospectively seems to have tilted the balance against them. Misadventure all the same!

What causes these accidents?

Human errors account for around 40 per cent and can arise from simple errors like entering a patient's blood group or allergies incorrectly in the file, to more complex errors like choosing and performing a wrong operation that proves overwhelming for the patient. Human errors are ubiquitous and occur in every organisation that depends on human beings, but their impact and consequences are never felt more than in the airlines and medical industries. The quality of recruits, their training, commitment, well-being (both professional and personal), monitoring, and supervision are key factors.

It is not difficult to observe how quality can be compromised at several levels. The recent media exposure of fraudulent pilots, who did not qualify through merit and did not receive adequate training, yet made their way into the airline industry sent shivers down our spine. The concern it generated probably stems from imagining ourselves on board a flight ten km up in the skies with the flight's controls in the hands of an untrained pilot, flying us to a collective doom. Human medical errors may not cause 'mass' deaths but 'serial' misadventures, some of which may turn fatal. In hospitals, disaster often strikes when the paths of an ill-fated patient and a careless overworked doctor cross.

Technical errors are the second most common. If you recount the last ten airline accident news reports, you will realise that most occurred due to technical snags with engines or systems letting them down; the Pawan Hans helicopter crashes are a case in point. Hospitals are no exception; despite locally feasible measures, malfunctions in hi-tech equipment do occur. Senior doctors point out that in the old days, medicine was ineffective but safe, whereas today's powerful treatments are effective but risky.

The third cause is organisational failure. The airline industry is much ahead in monitoring and tracking the quality of performance of all categories of its staff in an ongoing continuous mode, an area where hospitals are lagging far behind. The institutes of management and hospitals could work together and find solutions to some of these vexing problems.

08

Urinary Incontinence

In the journey of life, urinary incontinence may be a detour but it does not have to be the destination.

One of the reasons that keep some women away from outdoor activities and that they find embarrassing to discuss is urinary incontinence. Although not threatening to life, this disorder caused by a lack of control to hold back urine, often spoils the quality of life and makes it miserable.

Incontinence of urine is quite common; around ten per cent of adult women suffer from this disorder. The typical sufferer is a woman above 40, overweight, and had suffered an injury to the pelvic muscles while bearing children. The leakage of urine into undergarments or clothes is often intermittent during fits of coughing, sneezing, or while lifting heavy objects. It sometimes progresses to a state of constant dribbling.

The consequences are a feeling of being 'soiled' or a constant worry about it. Often the smell of urine can be a source of embarrassment in social gatherings that strong perfumes are unable to cover. She starts shying away from group activities, prefers to remain isolated, begins to lose self-esteem and often becomes depressed. The sense of leakage and soiling leads them to avoid sex.

The use of pads or STs helps provide temporary respite during travel and when going out for long periods. One can consider using it regularly, however, it can be expensive. Further, the constant feeling of being 'wrapped up' can hardly provide a sense of freedom or confidence in close interpersonal physical relationships, and one starts getting 'bound up' in spirits as well.

If one can come out of the initial inhibition and seek help, this disorder often responds well to treatment. The first step is to strengthen the muscles of the pelvis and the sphincter with exercises that a gynaecologist or urologist could teach. The weak muscular sphincter near the bladder neck gets strengthened and control returns. Medications to increase the tone of these muscles can also help provide early relief especially while waiting for the muscles to regain strength through exercise.

Few women with persistent incontinence require surgery. The pelvic muscles are tightened and a sling is passed around the urethra to restore control. This surgery is not risky but needs to be performed by an expert for good results.

Incontinence does occur in males as well but is less common. It usually follows surgery for the prostate. Sometimes it occurs when diabetes, surgery, or neurological diseases damage nerves that convey bladder sensation or impulses to sphincter muscles.

The satisfaction of feeling the fullness of the bladder, and keeping one's control on when and where to void urine is something we take for granted. Incontinence is a disruption of this fine control, that disrupts our social lives. Help is available as long as one is willing to overcome the initial embarrassment and seek it.

Section K

Technical Advances & Haunting Questions

Once you stop learning, you start dying. – Albert Einstein

01

Genetic Testing for Preventing Diseases

Knowing your genetic risk factors is like having a crystal ball for your health. It allows you to see into the future and take action to change the outcome.

With more people living longer, especially in cities, non-communicable diseases such as diabetes, heart disease, high blood pressure, depression, and cancer have now become new-age health problems. To keep pace with this changing landscape, research in medical science is throwing up new tools to detect risks and indicate protective strategies.

Yes, the age of genetic testing for personalised risk assessment and therapy is here. A Tennessee (USA) based laboratory, Mygenetx, and several others are providing just that. With a simple oral rinse, the laboratory can glean genetic information from the cells shed from the cheek and other data including age, weight, and lifestyle, providing you with a map to help you prevent health issues in the future.

It can tell you whether you have a genetic predisposition to developing diabetes, hypothyroidism, depression, hypertension, or heart disease. This information can be critical for, say an overweight person with a sedentary lifestyle. It could help him make decisions about his job, his daily schedule, his diet, and perhaps the frequency of monitoring his HbA1C levels.

Patients with diabetes interestingly fall into two categories: some have a variant of the haptoglobin gene called Hp2-2 and have a 500 per cent higher risk of heart attacks and strokes than those who do not have the variant. This information could be vital as a daily supplement taken by Hp2-2-positive diabetics could reduce their risk for heart disease and stroke to normal levels.

Genetic testing also helps identify people at risk for a variety of heart diseases such as aortic disorders, cardiomyopathy, arrhythmias, and many other structural heart problems. Many unexpected heart-related deaths, especially sudden deaths in young people, occur because of these disorders that go unrecognised. A positive genetic test could help cardiologists take a closer look to identify those more prone to potentially fatal rhythm disturbances and put them on medications before disaster strikes.

Depression is another common condition that often tends to slip through the fingers. It is an 'organic' disease in which the chemical neurotransmitters in the brain get out of balance. It runs in families, pointing to a genetic basis for it. Around 15 per cent of us are expected to suffer from depression in our lifetimes.

Genetic testing helps us know if we are predisposed. If one is, they could avoid stress-generating jobs, make adjustments to ensure more time with family and friends, and be alert to early recognisable symptoms. Recognising depression early helps shorten the period of suffering by initiating medicines early. Further, genetic testing could help determine which group of anti-depressant medications might be more suitable and in what doses, a clear example of the upcoming 'personalised medicine'.

The commercially available genetic tests can scan abnormalities in around 50 genes. It is humbling to remember that we have around 30,000 genes. Although a good beginning has been made, we still have a long way to go.

Fantasy, dreams, and science fiction do sometimes get transformed into reality, as recent developments in medical interventions are proving.

Up until the late eighties, surgery was synonymous with the use of the knife (surgeons call it scalpel to give it a distinctive status from the one used by butchers), large cuts or incisions, touching and handling of organs within the body, and cutting and sewing them according to need and intent.

Laparoscopic surgery, first developed by French surgeons, changed much of that tradition. Rather than making large cuts, they inserted longish instruments and imaging equipment into the body through small holes and operated without inserting their hands into the abdominal cavity. The outcomes were so spectacular in terms of shorter hospital stays, quicker recovery, reduced loss of blood, and much smaller scars, that the technique became popular across the world within two years.

It then became apparent that while few procedures, such as removal of the gallbladder, could be achieved by laparoscopic technique, many others such as cutting and removing deeper larger organs such as the pancreas or kidneys, still required the messy open route. Further, many organs, such as the prostate, are so deeply located in the pelvis, that getting to them with instruments or hands remains challenging.

This led to the development of robotic surgery, which uses robotic systems to overcome the limitations of pre-existing minimally invasive procedures.

Here, instead of directly moving the instruments, the surgeon uses a tele-manipulator that transmits his movements to the robotic arms that carry out the operation on the patient using end-effectors and manipulators. Typically, the surgeon is seated at a console a little away from the patient's bed, delves into a screen that provides him a three-dimensional view of the tissues, and blood vessels, and uses his hands and feet, as in a video game, to get the robot to carry out the surgery.

Robotic surgery provides better tissue dissection, more accurate surgery, less trauma, clear bloodless fields, and quicker recovery. The most popular instrument is the *da Vinci* system, more than 20 of which have already been installed in India and are functional.

A further refinement of robotic surgery is computer-assisted tele-surgery in which the operation can be performed by a surgeon from another city or continent, his movement being transmitted through computers to the robotic system.

If that is not sci-fi enough, watch out for the next quantum leap called cyberkinetic surgery. Here the surgeon does not have to use his hands to manipulate the controls, but can achieve it using sheer 'mental control'.

Remember how Yuri Geller from Israel, managed to bend spoons using mental powers alone? While some scientists ridiculed him and labelled him a fraud, several others followed up on what he claimed was possible. Scientists are now trying to develop systems where a surgeon can control the computer by his mental power or 'wish'.

Did this piece read like a bit of science fiction to you? Well, this is the rapidly changing realm of modern medical interventions.

02

How is 'Clean' Meat likely to be accepted by Vegetarians?

For vegetarians who have chosen their diet for ethical reasons, 'clean' meat provides a guilt-free option that respects their values while satisfying their desire for meat.

Many of us, especially in India, are wondering how the public will accept 'clean meat' which is hitting Western markets and likely to come to Indian markets by 2025.

To bring you on board on this topic, 'clean meat' or 'cultured meat' is real meat but grown in an artificial culture by tissue engineering. It is made from a few muscle cells or stem cells obtained from an animal by a needle, and made to multiply in the laboratory.

This is a new technology that is fast catching up, with several start-ups trying to grow meat by different methods. It, therefore, comes with fanciful names such as Memphis meat, based on the place or group. Scientists predict that very soon they will be able to grow around 50,000 kg of meat from just ten cells obtained from an animal, which does not have to be killed!

This technology promises to offer much. It would put a stop to the breeding and killing of animals, a concern that weighs heavily even on the hearts of some meat eaters. Further, it is likely to be environmentally friendly, freeing large stretches of land that are now used for grazing cattle. And is expected to reduce the production of greenhouse gases by almost 80 per cent.

In a world that is getting increasingly crowded and in which the environment is getting progressively murkier, one of the two transforming technologies that might bail humans out, could be this.

Cultured meat technology has followed the public imagination over the last few decades. Winston Churchill had said in 1931, possibly inebriatedly, "We shall escape the absurdity of growing a whole chicken to eat the breast or wing, by growing these parts separately under a suitable medium."

Initial costs have been predictably high. The first burger made and eaten in London in August 2013 came at a whopping cost of US$ 250,000 but is expected to match present prices of conventional meat and come down to just US$ 8.

The Australian bioethicist said, "Artificial meat stops cruelty to animals, is better for the environment, could be safer and more efficient, and even healthier. We have a moral obligation to support this kind of research. It gets the ethical two thumbs up." Animal welfare groups are generally in favour of the production of cultured meat because it does not have a nervous system and, therefore, cannot feel pain.

The question this technology will present is, *Would vegetarians be comfortable eating it? If not, Why?*

If cruelty and killing of animals is the primary concern for shunning animal meat, would this technology make vegetarians accept meat-eating?

For meat eaters, the appearance, taste, smell, and texture will also matter of course, but many will be morally relieved to eat meat without the burden of killing innocent animals weighing on their hearts.

This time around, traditions and religious texts won't help with the course of action but put us in the forefront to decide for ourselves.

03

Reproductive Science: Children with Three Parents

The birth of children with three biological parents underscores the ethical and moral questions that arise when science intersects with our fundamental notions of identity and family.

The latest salvo that reproductive biologists have fired at traditionalists since test-tube babies and surrogate motherhood has been the recent creation of babies with genetic material from three parents.

The scientific proof and benefits have been so compelling that the UK became the first country in the world to legalise it in 2015 despite several waves of protests and criticism from 'conventional' moralists.

Alan Saarinen is in her teens and looks and behaves like any other 'normal' schoolgirl of her age, playing sports and performing well in her class. She is, however, one of the rare 50 children in the world who has DNA from three parents: her father, mother, and a third lady who contributed mitochondria to fortify the defective egg of her mother.

Before she was born, her parents had tried for a baby for ten long years. Each time her mother Sharon had conceived through numerous IVF procedures, but the pregnancies had ended in spontaneous abortions or miscarriage.

It was then that the doctors discovered that Sharon carried a rare genetic trait due to which the mitochondria, the small power batteries of her ovum, were weak and defective. As a result, the embryo's organs that required generous amounts of oxygen, such as the heart, brain, and muscles, did not develop and function properly.

Dr. Jaques Cohen of New Jersey, USA, was the first to experiment with this technique that removes the cytoplasm containing the defective mitochondria of the diseased ovum and replaces it with normal mitochondria obtained from an ovum from a healthy donor woman. The 'corrected' ovum was then fertilised with the sperm in the laboratory as is done for test-tube babies.

While 90 per cent of DNA is present in the nucleus of human cells comprising 23,000 genes, small amounts comprising 15 genes are also present in mitochondria.

The potential of this technique was quickly recognised in the United Kingdom which has legalised it, but funnily the USA has withheld permission for this procedure at present. The concern of the American regulatory authorities and civil society is that formal permission may make this technique go down the unethical slippery slope of 'manufacturing' tailor-made babies in the laboratory.

New scientific developments in human reproductive biology always evoke sharp criticism and stiff resistance from ethics groups due to fear of potential misuse. Left to unscrupulous scientists, this technology can undoubtedly be used to produce made-to-order babies and in large amounts, almost like cloning animals.

But as of now, frustrated couples undergoing treatment for infertility in British clinics are looking forward to having their own babies with this technique.

04

Medical Boundaries and Life

In the face of illness and suffering, medical boundaries challenge us to seek innovative solutions while upholding the dignity of life.

An elderly neighbour passed away recently.

Of the many things we had on the long to-do list of the Sunday that comes just once a week, we kept pushing the unpleasant task of paying them a visit for a while before we took the plunge and knocked on their door.

The relatives wore a demeanour of sadness. Despite the initial uneasiness, they opened up to provide a vivid account of his ailments, sufferings, and treatments that he had been through over the last months.

For a brief while, the discussion did take that all too familiar route of when and how the doctor or hospital could have done that instead of this. I am not too sure whether it was because they knew me to be a doctor.

I refrained from getting sucked into a medical discussion and politely asked his age (it was 82), how long he had been ailing (two years), and what contributions and pleasant memories we had of him, the conversation bounced enthusiastically back to seeing death as an inevitable end to a glorious chapter of this gentleman's life and contributions.

His wife and son remarked how he had lived a full life, how his body had turned frail over the last two years as he suffered frequent bouts of pain, and how the curtain had to fall one day, one way or the other, on the day it did or perhaps on another day.

Despite our pride in being aware and 'knowledgeable', our acceptance of death as an inevitable 'natural' concluding chapter of living is still rather poor. We have learned to see it through the prism of reason and science. We still find it hard to accept that one may just die of old age, frail health, or the body just 'giving up' after eight decades of relentless service.

The legal definition of death is that the heart should have stopped beating irreversibly; we, therefore, often hunt for a respectable biomedical label such as cardiac failure, to convey that the heart indeed failed and stopped beating.

Every journey (by car, train, or air) has to come to an end, and so does life's journey, in death. It is, more often than not, a natural event, and learning to accept it makes life richer and provides it the grace it deserves.

Section L

Doctors as Humans

Wherever the art of medicine is loved, there is also a love of humanity. – Hippocrates

01

My Lesson in Endoscopy

As a medical practitioner, I am never tired of marvelling at the phenomenal achievements of science.

Armed with the latest, voluminous knowledge of diseases, diagnostic tests, drugs, and a few medical degrees, I had walked proudly into the world of medicine, My patient's symptoms and signs, laboratory reports and radiological findings, response to treatment and prognosis all seemed to so accurately fit what the medical textbooks described. And each year, the clinical experience strengthened my confidence in the latest state-of-the-art version of this wonderful science.

A frail, bedridden 83-year-old Mrs. Gehlaut had come to see three decades ago in my hey days. She was suffering from severe abdominal pain, jaundice, and fluctuating fever for some time. She was as apprehensive of my youth as I was of her old age. The duct through which bile flowed from her liver to the intestines was blocked and was converted into a bag of pus with stones. Since her chances of surviving a major surgery were slim, she had been advised to seek my help. It was not without trepidation that I confronted her with my offer of passing a rather thick endoscope down her throat to the intestines, passing an electric wire into the lower portion of her bile duct, and clearing the passage that was blocked with stones and pus. I did not mince words in explaining to her sons the considerable danger that the procedure carried in her vulnerable condition. The patient on her part seemed game.

With two of my juniors keeping a strict vigil on her pulse and respiration, two nurses assisting me with the instruments, and innumerable beads of perspiration breaking shamefully out on my forehead, I gently manoeuvred the tip of the endoscope past her vocal cords into her food pipe. Then it seemed to descend effortlessly down to her intestines as she lay relaxed and nodded in the affirmative when I asked her if all was well.

The cholangiography went off without any hitch and I inserted the electric knife into the lower end of the clogged bile duct. The knife was perfectly placed, and as I pressed on the footswitch the narrow opening slit open letting out a gush of pus and dirty bile into the gut. The procedure couldn't have been more perfect, I explained to the anxious relatives waiting outside. Several of her children, grandchildren, well-wishers, and friends looked admiringly at me as I explained with pride the complicated lifesaving feat that I had accomplished.

Mrs. Gehlaut went home the next day, feeling a lot better, and came back for a follow-up a month later with a big smile on her face having gained three kgs of weight. She had walked all the way to my office.

Encouraged by her mother-in-law's dramatic improvement at my hands, Rani came to consult me after being told that she had gallstones. She was around 40, young, pretty, and appeared a picture of perfect health and happiness. Her young son had just qualified in the recruitment exams of the defence services. Her problem was indeed a small one. The report of an ultrasound examination that she had undertaken mentioned that her bile duct was dilated possibly due to a small stone stuck at its lower end. The medical books recommend that such patients should have their stones removed via the endoscope or by surgery, the risk of serious complications with a wait-and-watch policy being unacceptably high. Foreseeing no problem, I proposed putting the same endoscope into her intestine just as I had for her mother-in-law and removing the offending small stone.

Rani smiled confidently as she walked up to the table. The procedure began with the usual precautions, and very soon the endoscope was sliding smoothly down Rani's food pipe and stomach to her duodenum. The mouth of the bile duct was easy to cannulate, and very soon we were taking pictures of the solitary small stone floating in it. I then asked for the electric wire knife as we prepared for the cut.

The wire knife did not slide into the bile duct easily. I changed the angle and tried again but it still did not work. I asked my assistant to administer an injection of a sphincter relaxant through the intravenous line and tried again, but did not succeed. I went on trying all the tricks I had learned during my training fellowships in Japan and Germany, but failure haunted me. My clothes were soaked in sweat when I finally gave up.

Barely half an hour later, Rani doubled up with severe pain. What I had feared did indeed happen—the stone moved to the lower end of the bile duct and obstructed the flow of bile. While we pumped antibiotics, painkillers, intravenous fluids, and hollow words of assurance into her, all night she tossed and groaned in agony and shivered as her temperature shot up to 105 F. By morning, she had jaundice.

Helplessness and guilt gnawed at me as I tried to confront her harassed relatives with scientific explanations.

I lay in bed soaked in shame and hurt, trying to rerun the events of the day in my mind, wondering where I had gone wrong. Why did this happen? To her? And to me? After wandering through the catacomb of logic and science without a meaningful answer, I began to realise there was perhaps something quite beyond my brain, my hands, and my skills. As the thick crusts of arrogance began peeling off my heart, I could hear the words of Ambroise Pare, a 16th-century French surgeon, echo in my ears: "I cleaned my patients' wounds and God healed them!"

FOLLOW-UP: After keeping us anxious for four days and teaching me the most important lesson in endoscopy, Rani's pain, fever, and jaundice settled as abruptly as it had started. She came to see me after a month when both of us agreed to let the sleeping stone lie. A year later, another ultrasound examination found her bile duct to be normal; the stone had passed out on its own! It made me feel rather small but by then I had learned to realise that I was indeed so and no bigger.

02

World Poetry Day and Medicine

Medicine and poetry share the common thread of empathy.
They both seek to understand and heal the human condition,
one through science, the other through verse.

In the rattle and jostle of news from the fields of politics, crime, and entertainment we gorge on daily, many of us fail to notice the coming and going of World Poetry Day on March 21.

Some of you might be preparing to 'switch off' right now, putting 'poetry' as a past-time, unconnected and distant from the rigid scientific realities of medicine and healthcare.

But then think again. Medicine is all about health, disease, fear, suffering, and sometimes death, and poetry happens to be the most powerful expression of emotion. Are we ignoring it at our own peril or stupidity?

First, for doctors who might be reading this piece—poetry is beginning to stand shoulder to shoulder with the jargon we use in scientific publications. Several reputed journals including the Lancet, the Journal of American Medical Association (JAMA), and The Annals of Internal Medicine accept and publish poems as they improve our understanding of human health and enhance HEALING.

Could we, therefore, be wearing blinkers while spouting technical terms in conferences and meetings, distancing ourselves from the real world of human perception and healing?

Second, several doctors have become the finest poets, such as John Keats, Arthur Conan Doyle, and Oliver Wendell Holmes to name a few. Their experience gave them the edge to feel and express emotions that only they could. I feel proud to belong to the same profession.

Third, poets can express suffering better than doctors can by capturing the feeling that is inseparably integrated with the clinical condition. Old age is not just about painful knees and wrinkling skin. TS Eliot wonderfully captures the spirit:

> 'I grow old… I grow old…
>
> I shall wear the bottoms of my trousers rolled.
>
> Shall I part my hair behind?
>
> Do I dare eat a peach?
>
> I shall wear white flannel trousers, and walk upon the beach.
>
> The mermaids are singing, each to each
>
> I do not think that they will sing to me.'

Last, but not least; the life, work, and attitude of a doctor needs to be inspiring, and we should remember that we are prone to the same sufferings and consequences that our patients go through.

Therefore, (quoting Langland)

> 'We should be low;
>
> and love-like, and lean each man to the other
>
> And patient as pilgrims,
>
> for pilgrims are we all.'

It was with ample reason that UNESCO dedicated a day to POETRY

03

Doctor, Banker, and a Dead Poet

A doctor's prescription heals the body, a banker's strategy secures the future, but a dead poet's verses nourish the heart.

On rare occasions, even medical consultations can turn interesting, as happened recently with a senior banker who had come to consult me for his stomach problem. As my list was not heavy that day, our discussion crossed the customary symptoms, sighs, and sorrows of bowel gas and constipation, funnily, to literature. He turned out to have been a student of English literature before becoming a banker. He couldn't hide his surprise that a medical specialist like me could be writing a weekly literary column for a newspaper for several years.

His surprise rose to astonishment when I proudly told him that at least five of the most celebrated writers he had pursued in college had come from my profession. My opening stroke began with Sir (Dr.) Arthur Conan Doyle, creator of the legendary Sherlock Holmes of 'The Hounds of Baskerville' fame. What enabled him to create that magical suspense was his deep knowledge of forensic medicine that he artfully meshed with a unique literary style, that evolved into matchless mystery stories sending shivers down the thickest of spines.

My next serve was Dr. W. Somerset Maugham, who had been my favourite during my high school days. His stories involved doctors, societies, and feelings. His ability to describe tumultuous human emotions and their conflicts remains unequalled and could inspire a generation of psychologists. His book, The Painted Veil, describes the emotional travails of a young doctor whose trauma of discovering his wife's unfaithfulness spurs him to risk his life and explore a dangerous epidemic, to which he succumbs, blurring the lines between valour and suicide. His semi-autobiography, Of Human Bondage, the story of a young child handicapped with a club foot who becomes a doctor, and the intricate interplay of his childhood frustrations, romantic obsessions, and acquired professional pleasure, remains a must-read for all literature lovers to this day.

The story of Dr. AJ Cronin, a Scottish doctor who turned into a celebrated novelist is also legendary. He was afflicted with tuberculosis soon after graduating from medical school, forcing him to rest for 6 months. Not having much to do, he took to writing; and so he became a very successful novelist with bestsellers such as The Citadel and The Stars Look Down that he never needed to practice medicine again. His writings deal with social themes viewed through the prism of a doctor.

Dr. Richard Gordon, famous for his 'Doctor' series (such as Doctor at Sea), scoops out humour from the lives of doctors that are usually filled with gory life-death stories. The funny anecdotes in his books can make even the most serious nuts break into a giggle, making many fellow passengers in airports and trains suspect the reader to have emerged from a loony bin.

We Indians, too, have had our share; the literary giant Balai Chand Mukhopadhya who wrote under the pen name, Banaphul, and produced immortal classics like 'Bhuban Shom' (remember the movie that won the Berlin award!), was a medical practitioner who wrote novels and stories when patients were few and far between.

Having proudly said all that, I challenged my banker patient to tell me if any from his profession had matched those from mine. He thought quietly for a while and admitted that he knew of only one banker, a despondent sardonic American poet named TS Eliot.

This time it was my turn to be stumped, as TS Eliot was indeed, ironically, my favourite modern poet, whose lyrical verses I have recited in times—good and bad!

Soon, my patient and I started seeing each other in a new light, as we began to recite Eliot together,

> *"We are the hollow men,*
> *We are the stuffed men,*
> *Leaning together,*
> *Headpiece filled with straw. Alas!"*

Sensing that something rather unusual was happening in the clinic that day, the nurse gingerly peeped to enquire if all was well, and whether I had discovered a long-lost relative. When I told her that we had just discovered a common favourite poet who bonded us, she scampered off more convinced than ever that we had both gone bonkers.

After a delightful hour, we brought our medical consultation to a close by reciting together the last stanza from Eliot's famous poem, probably the most quoted lines of any 20th-century English poetry:

> *'This is the way the world ends,*
> *This is the way the world ends,*
> *This is the way the world ends,*
> *Not with a bang,*
> *But with a whimper.'*

And retreated in Eliot's long shadow to our respective small lives of a doctor and a banker.

Epilogue: Trilogies of Health

The words 'Health' and 'Disease' evoke widely differing responses and emotions, from eating an apple daily on the one hand to suffering heart attacks on the other. A good starting point is taking a closer look at health, not merely as the absence of a serious disease but as physical, mental, emotional, and social well-being. It is broad and goes well beyond the body, embracing mental and psychosocial aspects too. The vital mind-body connection, disregarded for decades, has been finally endorsed by scientific bodies across the world.

Healthy living cannot be found at the chemist's shop, the gymnasium, or the spa. Each one of us has to decide what our needs are to make living as healthy a journey as we possibly can.

It, therefore, needs a perspective as we go on this time-bound journey called life and take a look at our bodies, our minds, and our reactions to the environment and circumstances we come across during the journey.

Though we see the same world, we see it through different eyes.
– Virginia Woolf

Life-health-living-happiness-disease-death form a continuum that we cannot wish away. We often obsess about a narrow physical aspect at the cost of a larger 'bio, psycho, social, and philosophical' approach. This book, the first of two volumes, aims to acquaint the reader with the BIO or physical issues and provide a perspective on how they can be seen in the larger context of a well-lived life.

Health is a part of three trilogies.

Trilogy 1. Knowledge-Attitude-Practice/Behaviour (KAP)

The first bead of the KAP trilogy is, of course, **knowledge** or awareness, which is usually accepted as the starting point in an educated society.

When you fear something, learn as much about it as you can. Knowledge conquers fear. – Edmund Burke

Knowledge does help dispel the fear that the thought of illness or the uncertainty of health brings to our minds. It is never too early or too late to start familiarising yourself with the common conditions, many of which we encounter as we go through life.

The second is **attitude**—how we wear that knowledge on our sleeves as we walk through life. An example of the discrepancy between knowledge and attitude is when we know something, such as the harmful effects of smoking, yet continue to smoke because it looks 'cool'. Attitude is shaped by several factors apart from knowledge, with societal and cultural practices and peer pressures chipping in.

Behaviour or **practice** is the third bead; how do our knowledge and attitude translate into behaviour? We may know the potential benefits of keeping our weight in check, but are we able to set and achieve lifestyle goals with diet and regular exercise?

Trilogy 2: Living and Well-being-Disease-Death

We are conditioned to conveniently forget that life is lent to us for a limited period, and it would be most unusual not to encounter hurdles during the journey. As one stage merges into the next—childhood, adolescence, adulthood, middle and then old age in imperceptible ways, disruptions or diseases come and go quite as the norm rather than exceptions. This book is like a casual travelogue that deals with some of the common ones you might encounter on the journey.

Life can only be understood backwards, but it must be lived forwards. – Soren Kierkegaard

Observing and learning early could be advantageous.

Trilogy 3: Existence-Purpose-Happiness

The third trilogy may, at first, seem over the head, but poses questions about purpose and meaning that every conscious person may need to ask and try to answer.

The mystery of human existence lies not just in staying alive but having something to live for. – Fyodor Dostoevsky

I have observed many patients come to consult me about minor issues, such as a slightly lower reading of vitamin D in their blood profile, but are unmindful of the directionless and unhappy life they are leading.

Most humans need a sense of purpose to keep going through life. Many believe the goal should be 'happiness'; some use other expressions such as fulfilment or satisfaction of a journey well traversed and a destination gracefully reached.

A good amount of ongoing research from several parts of the world is trying to understand 'happiness', beyond just a pleasant mood or good feeling, to a deeper understanding of this positive state of mind, and its relationship to health and well-being.

As you might have realised by now, health is a nebulous topic that encompasses many ideas. This book hopes to provide a deeper (but not detailed) perspective on this broad issue, stimulate you to think beyond the elementary do's and don'ts, and provide a simplified version of a series of medical topics.

Hope some portions of the book, if not all of it, will enhance your insight, tickle your emotions, and stimulate new thought.

www.ingramcontent.com/pod-product-compliance
Lightning Source LLC
LaVergne TN
LVHW041151150826
845673LV00001B/134

* 9 7 9 8 8 9 0 6 7 7 1 4 3 *